A. Lerner · D. Reis · M. Soudry

Severe Injuries to the Limbs

A. Lerner · D. Reis · M. Soudry

Severe Injuries to the Limbs

Staged Treatment

With 804 Figures, Mostly in Colour

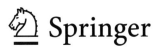 Springer

Alexander Lerner, MD
Daniel Reis, MD
Michael Soudry, MD

Department Orthopaedic Surgery
Rambam Health Care Campus
Faculty of Medicine
Technion, Israel Institute of Technology
Haifa, 31096, Israel

Library of Congress Control Number: 2006940072

ISBN   978-3-540-69892-0   Springer Berlin Heidelberg New York

Springer-Verlag is a part of Springer Science+Business Media
springer.com

Editor: Gabriele Schröder, Heidelberg, Germany
Desk Editor: Irmela Bohn, Heidelberg, Germany
Reproduction, typesetting and production: LE-TEX Jelonek, Schmidt & Vöckler GbR, Leipzig, Germany
Cover design: Frido Steinen-Broo, EStudio, Calamar, Spain

Printed on acid-free paper   24/3180/YL 5 4 3 2 1 0

3/20/08

This book is dedicated to our wives Galina Lerner,
Batsheba Rosental-Reis, and Esther Soudry,
without whose understanding and support
it would not have seen the light of day.

Foreword

Polytrauma is a disease of our modern high-speed society. Most cities have designated trauma centers that administer to individuals with multiple injuries. Most trauma centers are not prepared, trained or equipped to treat the severity of injuries or number of patients that present from terrorist or war trauma. This book presents an authoritative organized comprehensive approach to orthopedic war injuries of bone and soft tissues. Dr. Alexander Lerner is one of the foremost authorities in the world in this field, working at Rambam Hospital in Haifa, where geo-political circumstances have delivered civilians and military personnel injured at war or from terrorism to the hospital's doors. While various fixation methods are presented, innovative methods using external fixation are the centerpiece of this book. Some of these techniques provide orthopedic surgeons with methods to avoid the need for extensive plastic surgery procedures by using the external fixators' abilities to reposition the bone fragments. The techniques of bone transport, fracture and nonunion distraction as well as various soft-tissue reconstruction methods are discussed, illustrated, and taught in detail.

This book is an essential guide for today's trauma centers that deal with urban warfare and for many urban hospitals and orthopedic trauma surgeons that may be called upon to treat mass casualties due to accidents or terrorism. Military surgeons will use this tome as a guide book for the treatment and reconstruction of war-injured patients. This unique book is the unfortunate product of our insecure world but by the same token is essential for the survival of those unfortunate enough to be traumatized in today's world conflicts. This book is well written and illustrated with numerous photographs, radiographs and illustrations.

Dror Paley, MD, FRCSC
Director of the Rubin Institute for Advanced
Orthopedics at Sinai Hospital of Baltimore
Co-Director
The International Center for Limb Lengthening
Sinai Hospital of Baltimore
2401 West Belvedere Avenue
Baltimore, Maryland 21215, USA

Preface

The treatment of severe locomotor system trauma has a long tradition in our hospital, the Rambam Medical Center, Haifa, the only tertiary hospital in the north of Israel covering a population of almost 2 million citizens. Our hospital lies less than 20 min helicopter flying time from the border, and hence, sadly due to the ever-present outbreaks of war and terror in the north of Israel along the Lebanese and Syrian borders, our trauma and orthopedic teams have accumulated vast experience in the treatment of severe injuries of the musculoskeletal system. As the major referral center for all the hospitals in the north of the country, the orthopedic and trauma departments take in civilian and military patients suffering from complex primary or secondary orthopedic trauma.

This book summarizes the authors' accumulated experience in the treatment of severe wounds of the limbs. The constant stream of major military and civilian trauma has afforded us the opportunity to develop our staged method. Without exception, all the cases reported in this book that demonstrate our staged treatment are taken from our own archives.

Sophisticated techniques for the care of massive injuries to the soft tissues and the most modern devices and methods for the fixation of severe fractures have been integrated into our treatment protocols. The staged treatment protocol, based on minimally invasive external fixation and the biological principles of tissue reconstruction by distraction tissue genesis (the versatile Ilizarov technique), permits the reconstruction of severely injured limbs and at the same time avoids serious complications.

In this monograph we report on the accumulated experience of 40 years in the treatment of severe injuries of the musculoskeletal system with grave tissue loss, and in particular war injuries. Emphasis is given to the proper attention and care of the soft tissues, sequential damage control, and the judicious staged use of appropriate external fixation.

The authors wish to thank and pay tribute to the relentless day and night work of all the devoted surgeons and nurses who have participated in the care of our patients over the years; in particular, the residents, senior orthopedic surgeons, and previous and current heads of the orthopedic departments at Rambam Medical Centre, without whose devotion and dedication this work could not have been done. We wish, in particular, to pay a special tribute to Professor Haim Stein, Emeritus Associate Professor, and former director of the Department of Orthopedic Surgery A. Professor Stein promoted, stimulated, and himself took part in limb salvage surgery until his retirement. He deserves much credit for the evolution of our staged method of treatment which depends so much on the principles of external fixation.

In conclusion, we hope that this book will be helpful to orthopedic, trauma and military surgeons treating severe high-energy limb trauma, especially limb salvage in severe war injuries, and elective limb reconstruction surgery and rehabilitation. We dedicate this book to our patients, without whose courage, fortitude, and motivation to be rehabilitated, our attempts would not have been successful.

Alexander Lerner
Senior Lecturer

Daniel Reis
Emeritus Associate Clinical Professor

Michael Soudry
Associate Clinical Professor and Chairman

Division of Orthopedic Surgery
Rambam Health Care Campus
Faculty of Medicine
Technion, Israel Institute of Technology
Haifa, Israel

Contents

Introduction

In recent decades, the number of injuries caused by high-energy trauma has increased significantly due to the greater number of severe road traffic accidents, work trauma, and also firearm and blast injuries due to local military conflicts and terror attacks. More than 75% of all injuries in modern warfare are to the extremities, with a high risk of deep wound infection and post-traumatic osteomyelitis (caused by free bone fragments stripped of their periosteum), severe covering-tissue defects, and concomitant vascular injuries [16]. In recent local regional conflicts, there were relatively fewer thoracic and abdominal injuries but more damage to the extremities, due to the use of body protective vests. In road traffic accidents, modern safety equipment, such as seat belts and airbags, has changed the pattern of injuries, protecting the head and vital organs of the trunk. However, the extremities, especially the lower ones, are exposed to injury, and often suffer complex fractures [86, 135]. The number of multi-trauma patients reaching emergency rooms alive has increased, thanks to the fact that more emergency medical and paramedic teams are trained to cope with life-threatening critical conditions, and due to the rapid evacuation of battlefield casualties and victims of terror attacks to trauma centers that provide the required care immediately.

High-energy injuries to the limbs, involving both bone and soft tissue, remain complex injuries to treat, especially when associated with life-threatening injuries [2]. This is highly relevant to war injuries, especially blast injuries, which, by their high-energy impact, cause extensive blunt soft-tissue injury due to the blast wave, multiple penetrating fragment injuries, heavy contamination of the tissues, and a high rate of compartment syndrome. According to Nechaev et al. [99], most of the injuries in the Afghanistan war were multiple and complex (59.4%–72.8%), and more than half the injured were admitted in severe and critical condition. The management of open fractures is challenging, and multiple complex surgical procedures are frequently needed to achieve soft-tissue coverage, fracture union, and restoration of function [146].

Traditionally, firearm injuries have been divided into high- and low-velocity categories, based on projectile muzzle velocity. Low-velocity missile wounds are more common in the civilian population, and are typically caused by projectiles with a muzzle velocity of less than 610 m/s or 2000 ft/s (mostly handguns). They cause less tissue destruction and generally the injury can be treated after wound excision by closed fracture principles. Tissue damage is usually more substantial with higher velocity weapons (more than 610 m/s or 2000 ft/s) [4]; for example, injuries caused by modern military rifles and mine blasts. In modern local wars, more and more wounds are caused by splinters due to blast injuries (63.4%–73.5% of the injuries in the Afghanistan war, according to Nechaev et al. [99]). Wounding potential and lethality are related to the amount of kinetic energy that the projectile is able to impart to the target. Kinetic energy can be expressed by the formula: $KE = (m \cdot v^2)/2$, where m is mass and v is velocity.

Tissue damage is proportional but not equal to the amount of kinetic energy deposited in the target, calculated by subtracting the amount of kinetic energy of the bullet on exit from the amount of kinetic energy on impact with the body. Although a projectile's velocity and mass are inseparable, a greater mass results only in a linear increase in kinetic energy, whereas a change in velocity affects energy exponentially to the second power [5]. The bullet velocity is a major determining factor in the production of tissue damage [86]. The greater velocity leads to magnified energy absorption, which leads to increased tissue damage [35]. Commonly, gunshot wounds in civilians (low-velocity missiles) have more focal injury patterns and usually cause limited tissue damage from the missile injury alone, and not from cavitation effects [42, 59]. The majority of patients with low-velocity gunshot wounds may be safely and economically treated non-operatively with simple local wound care (superficial irrigation and careful dressing, with or without antibiotics) on an outpatient level, while associated limb fractures can be stabilized according to the principles in use for closed limb fractures, because of their similar characteristics (but see reservations below) [3, 5, 12, 59]. Modern military high-velocity missiles produce significant cavitations and fragments during their terminal ballistic phase. If the missile strikes bone, fragmentation of the bone, of the missile, or both may occur, and the resultant secondary missiles will produce additional tissue damage [34]. Gunshot wounds and blast injuries can cause either penetrating (not exiting) or perforating (exiting) wounds. The radiological appearance of a foreign body in the tissue of an injured limb is clear evidence that all the contained kinetic energy was expended in the missile–tissue interaction. Fragmentation of bullets has also been reported to correlate with higher missile velocity and delivered energy [36]. According to Gugala and Lindsey [42], the extent of bone comminution corresponds directly to the amount of missile energy transferred, and also suggests the degree of soft-tissue injury. In contrast, only some of the kinetic energy is absorbed by the tissues in perforating wounds where bullets fragments are not detected on radiography. Limited energy transfer by high-velocity missiles produces relatively less tissue damage and, in contrast, efficient transfer of energy by low-velocity missiles can result in devastating wounds [5]. Moreover, the impact energy of low-velocity shotguns at close range is similar to that of high-velocity firearms. Therefore, simply designating gunshot injuries as low-velocity or high-velocity wounds alone does not accurately reflect the true extent of the injury severity [42]. More appropriate and more important than velocity are the designations "low-energy" and "high-energy" which are more descriptive of the extent of tissue damage. Moreover, according to Long et al. [88], who studied the accuracy of classification systems for gunshot injuries in civilians, they do not provide a true description of the weapons because more than one-quarter of patients who suffered from firearm injuries cannot identify the weapon and, in many patients, the description is unreliable. He concluded that, in deciding upon treatment without knowing the type of weapon, the clinical and radiological appearance of the injured limb dictates the treatment protocol, and patients with extensive devitalized wounds must be treated according to the protocol for patients suffering from high-energy injuries.

The condition of the soft tissue of the injured limb is a vital factor, determining the chances of limb salvage procedures and the feasibility of functional restoration. In these fractures, the injuring agent transfers significant energy to the soft-tissue envelope, traumatizing these vulnerable structures and increasing the risk of major complications. Therefore, the initial care must be minimally traumatic and maximally sparing of the already damaged soft tissues. All fractures should be stabilized as early as possible. These patients are often polytraumatized and hypotensive, and may be hypothermic and coagulopathic. The use of a temporary external fixation device allows adequate resuscitation of the patient prior to definitive fixation [47]. High-energy trauma can include neurosurgical, general surgical, maxillo-facial, ophthalmologic, otolaryngological, inhalation, burns, and other injuries. Rapid skeletal stabilization in patients with multiple complex fractures allows resuscitation with minimal blood loss and operative time [47], affording time for additional diagnostic imaging and adequate preoperative planning for the definitive elective limb reconstruction. The complexity and variability of these injuries dictate that routine prescriptive management based on fixed protocols is not possible and, therefore, a flexible and individualized approach to treatment is required [63].

Even in patients who suffer from closed fractures, soft-tissue injury plays a central role in prognosis and management. Because of the possibility of further soft-tissue damage caused by unstable fractures, the main bone fragments must be stabilized without delay. Stability is a very important factor, especially when there is a combined injury. Unstable fractures cause pain, nursing problems, morbidity, and mortality. Impaired bone healing results in delayed union or even nonunion. In contrast, early and sufficient fracture stabilization improves the recovery of the overlying soft tissues and the fracture itself. This is especially so in the treatment of patients suffering from war injuries, because the great forces involved result in extensive destruction of the bone and surrounding soft-tissue envelope. Classical fixation methods of fractures, such as plaster of Paris casting and continuous skeletal traction, are not acceptable in the treatment of patients suffering from high-energy unstable fractures with severely compromised soft tissues. Massive soft-tissue damage, extensive wounds (including post-fasciotomy wounds), and extensive post-traumatic fracture blisters require intensive daily soft-tissue care and preclude the use of cast immobilization. Furthermore, such severe fractures would require a relatively long period of immobilization, and this would result in stiffness in the neighboring joints. In addition, cast fixation cannot provide sufficient stability for early weight-bearing in patients with comminuted high-energy fractures, especially with bone loss. Skeletal traction, demanding lengthy immobilization, is unacceptable for treating patients with multiple and combined injuries, who require early mobilization and active nursing care.

Heavy contamination of the injured tissues precludes the use of internal fixation methods for fracture stabilization in these patients. Interlocking intramedullary fixation provides stabilization, achieved without additional periosteal damage, with secure control of alignment and rotation of bone fragments, wide access for soft-tissue care, early mobilization of the patient, and early movement of the adjacent joints. Interlocking nails have become the treatment of choice in the management of diaphyseal fractures of the long bones, including many types of open fractures. The disadvantages of this method are the potential spread of infection throughout the medullary canal along the nail, hardware failure due to the relatively small nail size, and technical difficulties in the treatment of distal and proximal one-third fractures. A study by Henley et al. [53] demonstrated a slight advantage of the unreamed interlocking intramedullary nail over unilateral 5.0-mm half-pin external fixators in the treatment of Gustilo Type II, IIA, and IIIB open fractures of the tibial shaft. However, patients with the most complex injuries, such as Gustilo Type IIIC fractures, tibial fractures caused by firearm projectiles, and fractures with significant bone loss, were excluded from this study, thereby significantly affecting its results.

Reamed interlocking intramedullary nails have a mechanical advantage over unreamed nails, but the reaming procedure of long tubular bones causes both mechanical and thermal damage to the medullary blood supply which cannot be tolerated when the injury has stripped much of the periosteal blood supply from the bone. According to Melcher et al. [94], reaming of the medullary cavity with the attendant reduction in local vascularity and necrosis may be additional risk factors.

The method of fracture stabilization utilizing a standard plating technique requires extensive tissue dissection. Exposure of the fracture site and bone fragments should be limited, in order to retain vascularization. A precondition for performing the plating procedure is the availability of immediate and reliable coverage of the fracture site and implanted internal fixator by viable soft tissues, and this condition is frequently absent in war injuries. The concept of "biological fixation" with new plate designs and minimized bone-plate contact, bridge-plating techniques, and improved surgical techniques with percutaneously inserted plates has led to improved rates of fracture union and a decreased incidence of infection and other postoperative complications. However, even the limited local pressure of plates on bone can damage the blood supply, essential for fracture healing, to the underlying bone [50]. Furthermore, an implanted internal fixator foreign body promotes infection in the wound in cases of septic complications. Even limited contact pressure plates require safe soft-tissue coverage without any compromise. Incisions through compromised tissue can lead to wound breakdown and deep infection [135]. Thus, methods of internal fixation using intramedullary nails or plating provide fracture stabilization at the cost of disturbing the intramedullary or periosteal blood supply [19]. Based on his experience in treating war injuries to the extremities, Busic et al. [16] reported a high rate of deep infection (33%) when internal fixation was used as the primary management. Hence, an internal fixator should not be used as a method of choice in the initial stages of treatment of war injuries. Long et al. [88] observed 100 patients who underwent surgical treatment for civilian gunshot injuries to the femur. They found that the femoral fractures

of 79 patients with minimal soft-tissue damage united without infection, but 8 of 21 patients with severe soft-tissue damage had deep infection.

Fracture healing depends on an adequate blood supply and sufficient stability of fixation for a successful end result. The severity of the soft-tissue injury rather than the choice of implant appears to be the predominant factor influencing rapidity of bone healing and rate of injury site infection [53].

In treating poly-traumatized patients, external fixation provides a quick and minimally invasive approach. Using external fixation as a more biological method of skeletal stabilization helps preserve tissue vascularity. The advantages of this extra-focal method of fixation also include retention of the fracture hematoma without disturbing the soft-tissue envelope at the fracture site. Using external fixation frames in the management of these patients allows both quick stabilization and realignment of shattered bones, with minimal surgical invasion and additional disruption of the mangled soft tissue. The principle behind this method is stabilization of fracture fragments by the combination of transfixion of fracture fragments and an external stable framework distanced from the wound and capable of repeated adjustments [147]. There is no need for insertion of massive foreign bodies (internal fixators) into the fracture zone, demanding an appropriate surgical approach with additional incisions and soft-tissue trauma, in addition to adequate soft-tissue coverage of the bone ends, fracture zone, and implanted internal fixators. Care must be taken not to add further surgical devascularization of the bone ends. Thus, fracture stabilization is achieved without further compromising the already damaged soft-tissue envelope. External fixation frames allow simple and quick bone stabilization, provide simplicity in nursing care, and allow earlier mobilization of patients. The wounds are easily accessed and local treatments, including necessary surgical procedures, are readily applied. This versatile method of treatment may be employed in almost any configuration, severity, and localization of fracture. Reduction and stabilization of bone fragments should be performed with minimal trauma to the tissues, avoiding additional dissection, stripping and iatrogenic devascularization of the bone fragments (*primum non nocere*). Methods of external fixation, techniques using indirect fracture reduction, and procedures that obviate the need for direct exposure of the fracture site can avoid some of the complications associated with open reduction and internal fixation of bone fragments. According to Efimenko et al. [32], the introduction of functionally stable external osteosynthesis improves the results of treatment of gunshot limb fractures. External skeletal fixation is the preferred initial treatment for stabilizing severe open missile fractures of the limbs, reducing the rate of morbidity and limb amputations [47, 140].

Modern external fixation equipment is relatively easy to use and teach. It achieves quick, effective, primary fracture stabilization. These important properties are suited to operations, often executed under emergency conditions by duty teams of orthopedic residents, in the absence of highly skilled specialists in the field of limb salvage and reconstruction.

Temporary external fixation has been recommended to provide relative bone stability while the soft tissue heals, prior to formal open reduction and internal fixation. According to Haidukewych [47], using a protocol of temporary external fixation in complex peri-articular fractures will allow time to prepare the patient for surgery, prepare the surgeon for what needs to be done, and prepare the injured extremity for surgery. The use of temporary external fixation is an attractive strategy in the staged treatment of complex fractures.

External fixation devices provide several important advantages:
- Extra-focal fixation technique;
- Relatively easy application technique;
- Rapid and relatively stable fracture fixation using a minimal number of parts;
- Adequate fixation frame for any fracture configuration;
- Low morbidity, minimally invasive fixation technique;
- Temporary trans-articular bridging can be performed in patients with severe intra- and juxta-articular injuries.

The main disadvantages of external fixation are:
- Require daily pin-tract care;
- Discomfort;
- Local pin-tract infection rate;
- Sometimes interference with soft-tissue reconstruction;
- Muscle transfixion can result in neighboring joint stiffness;
- Need for prolonged on-going orthopedic follow-up in an outpatient clinic.

Primary Treatment

2

2.1 Primary Treatment and "Damage Control"

Patients who present with associated life-threatening injuries should be evaluated and resuscitated according to Advanced Trauma Life Support protocols. The initial care of a massively traumatized limb begins with the resuscitation of the patient, especially in patients suffering from multiple trauma. Surgical damage control includes an operative technique in which control of bleeding and stabilization of vital signs become the priority in saving the patient, together with prevention of contamination and protection from further injury. Severe multiple injuries can initiate a cascade of events resulting from blood loss and release of inflammatory mediators, leading to a "vicious cycle" of shock, hypothermia, acidosis, and coagulopathy, resulting in end-organ failure and death [51, 91]. Damage-control surgery is the most technically demanding and challenging surgery a trauma surgeon can perform. Many studies have reported that immediate stabilization of long bone fractures drastically reduced adult respiratory distress syndrome (ARDS), multiple organ failure (MOF), and sepsis – the effect of the "golden 24 h" [86]. The more severe the injury, the greater the effect of early fracture stabilization. Sufficient bone stabilization allows early mobilization from the bed, preventing severe complications, such as pneumonia and thromboembolic disease. The presence of major fractures increases the risk of MOF syndromes. This risk can be reduced by a comprehensive plan for early management, including operative fracture stabilization. However, the poly-trauma patient who survives the "first hit" from the trauma itself must be protected from the "second hit" phenomenon, i.e., the results of traumatic surgery.

Pape et al. [105] investigated the impact of intramedullary nailing as opposed to temporary external fixation for the treatment of femoral fractures in severely injured patients. In this study, an attempt was made to determine the operative burden by evaluating the perioperative concentrations of pro-inflammatory cytokines (interleukin-1, interleukin-6, and interleukin-8) in central venous blood. A significant and sustained inflammatory response was measured after intramedullary nailing performed within 24 h, but not after initial external fixation. These findings suggest that damage-control orthopedic surgery minimized the additional physiological impact induced by acute intramedullary fixation of the femur.

The concept of damage control orthopedics (DCO), relative to limb surgery in patients with severe multiple injuries, is an attempt to minimize the "second hit" of an emergency procedure of long bone stabilization, performed rapidly and atraumatically, and to release compartment syndromes. The principles of DCO are used to reduce the degree of surgical impact on patients with severe multiple injuries who are at risk for MOF. Vital for achieving this goal are minimizing the duration of initial surgery, avoiding additional blood loss, and performing only life- and limb-saving procedures [51] (Fig. 2.1.1).

2.2 Tissue Debridement

Often, the first surgical procedure determines the long-term outcome of severe trauma. Major organ trauma may be present in patients suffering from high-energy, especially war, injuries. After stabilization of the patient's general condition, a thorough head-to-toe examination must be performed, checking the blood supply to the limbs, the neurological status of the limb, the bony stability, and the soft-tissue condition of injured extremities. Each wound should be evaluated completely and treated appropriately. It is essential to examine more than just the wound area; the entire extremity must be evaluated and radiographs of the adjacent joints must be obtained [5]. Radiographs of the fracture help determine the energy of the injury, although the soft-tissue damage is usually greater than what is visually evident [144]. Tetanus prophylaxis should be administered immediately, based on the patient's immunization status. Intravenous antibiotic combination therapy [115] using a first-generation cephalosporin (cefazolin 1.0 g t.i.d.) active against Gram-positive organisms, and an aminoglycoside (gentamicin 240 mg/day), active against Gram-negative organisms, is started in the emergency room

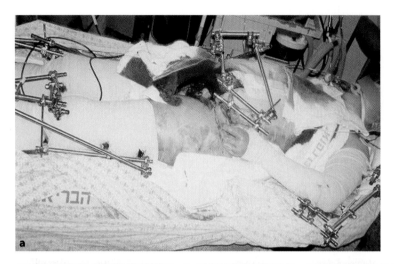

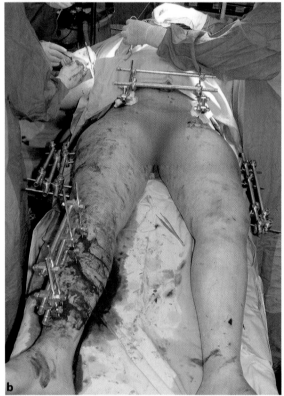

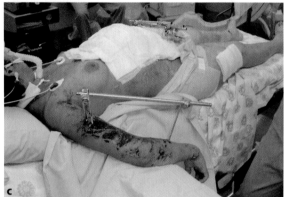

Fig. 2.1.1a–c. Primary external skeletal stabilization used in emergency treatment of complex poly-trauma patients

for patients suffering from open combat trauma and is continued for 3 days. Penicillin 5,000,000 units q.i.d. should be added to the antibiotic regimen when conditions favoring the development of anaerobic infections exist (soil contamination and vascular injuries). As soon as the patient is hemodynamically stable, he or she must be taken to the operating room.

The major factor determining the outcome in high-energy injuries to the limbs is the severity of the soft-tissue injury. Open fractures communicate with the outside environment and the resulting contamination of the wound with microorganisms, coupled with the compromised vascular supply to the region, leads to an increased risk of infection as well as to complications in healing [146]. Primary radical debridement is a crucial phase in the management of patients after open high-energy injuries. Aggressive extensive debridement of all damaged tissue surrounding the bullet tract from high-velocity military weapons has been standard military surgical practice. Inadequate debridement remains the major cause of chronic infection after severe extremity trauma [130]. In 2003, Bartlett wrote: "The evaluation and treatment of damaged muscle remains one of the surgeon's greatest challenges" [4]. Inadequate debridement of open fractures is often the rule rather than the exception, because tissue devitalization is usually not appreciated immediately [22, 45, 108, 129]. Inadequate excision of missile wounds of the extremities will leave necrotic tissue in the wound, predisposing to infection and to possible later amputation [148]. No principle is more important in the care of an open fracture than copious irrigation and meticulous wound debridement [141]. Before the patient is anesthetized, a thorough neurological examination of the injured limb should be conducted, unless the patient is unconscious, or a proximally placed tourniquet is in place, creating limb numbness.

General anesthesia is the "gold standard" for the treatment of patients suffering from multiple fractures to the limbs. Spinal or regional anesthesia can be useful tools for treating patients with isolated damage to the limbs.

Thorough and copious irrigation of contaminated wounds will lower the risk of infection [102]. However, there is no consensus regarding optimal volume, pressure, or the desirable additives to the irrigation fluid [59]. According to a study performed by Draeger and Dahners [29], suction and sharp debridement, as practiced by most surgeons, may remove foreign bodies well without the use of high-pressure pulsatile lavage (HPPL). Moreover, HPPL may drive some contaminants deeper into tissue already compromised by trauma, rather than remove them. Furthermore, this study supports the conclusion that pulsatile lavage rather than low-pressure irrigation methods, including bulb syringe and suction irrigation, may further damage soft tissues.

In performing a primary debridement procedure, the involved limb is prepared circumferentially and draped free so as to leave all important skeletal landmarks visible. A tourniquet is applied to the proximal part of the extremity, to be used only when necessary (active bleeding); otherwise, the debridement procedure is completed without inflating the tourniquet. This prevents additional ischemic damage to already severely traumatized tissues during the operative procedure. In addition, there may have been a prolonged tourniquet time from the injury event until hospital admission. Even when a tourniquet is obligatory, the tourniquet time should be kept to a minimum, since using a tourniquet in treating lower extremity trauma has been shown to increase the incidence of wound infection, presumably by increasing tissue hypoxia and acidosis [112].

Generally, the operation is performed with repeated and thorough washing of the post-traumatic wound and skin on all surfaces of the injured extremity with chlorhexidine soapy scrub followed by normal saline and/or Ringer's solution. An additional flushing with hydrogen peroxide solution is recommended. All visible and palpated foreign bodies must be removed from the wound. All devitalized soft tissues in the wound bed must be removed. The denuded and comminuted bone fragments with questionable viability must also be removed. Wounds are surgically extended into the adjacent "normal" tissues along the lines of described surgical exposure to allow for complete visualization and adequate exposure of the tissues in the trauma zone. Primary surgical debridement of the wound must be radical and aggressive, with excision of all devitalized tissues which can be a source of tissue necrosis and infection in the future. Excision of the wound skin edges not only removes devitalized tissues but also improves the exposure of the depth of the wound.

The borders of the damaged tissue area with the normal tissues in cases of high-energy trauma are usually contused and can not be precisely distinguished. The classic symptoms of the "four Cs" – color, consistency, contractility, and the capacity to bleed continuously – must be checked and detected during surgical debridement of muscle [4]. When the borders have been defined, all non-viable skin, subcutaneous fat, and muscle should be removed sharply. All intact segmental muscular vascular branches must be preserved to avert further local muscle ischemia. All non-viable tissue must be removed, while as much functional tissue of the tendons, joint capsule, and ligaments as possible is spared during extensive debridement unless it is extremely contaminated or macerated (Fig. 2.2.1).

Debridement of non-viable soft tissue and irrigation with normal saline are repeated during the operative procedure. All denuded bone fragments must be removed from the wound, avoiding devascularization of the fracture zone. According to Brusov et al. [14], a 5- to 5.5-cm degloving of the periosteum from the bone ends can be detected in most cases of high-energy trauma. Bony debridement is controversial, with recommendations varying from replacing large free contaminated cortical fragments to removing cortical bone until bleeding from the edges is seen [92]. The fragments are most often saved to add to the mechanical integrity of internal fixation. According to McAndrew and Lantz [92], deep wound infection occurred in 7%–25% of patients in whom devascularized cortical fragments were saved, and these failures were commonly due to inadequate bone debridement. The various possibilities of the Ilizarov method in providing stable fixation in patients with severe bone comminuting, even in cases of extensive post-traumatic bone loss, and the potential bridging of bone defects using distraction osteogenesis, allows for radicalism during primary surgical debridement. This reduces the quantity of non-vital tissues in the wound, thus diminishing the risk of wound deterio-

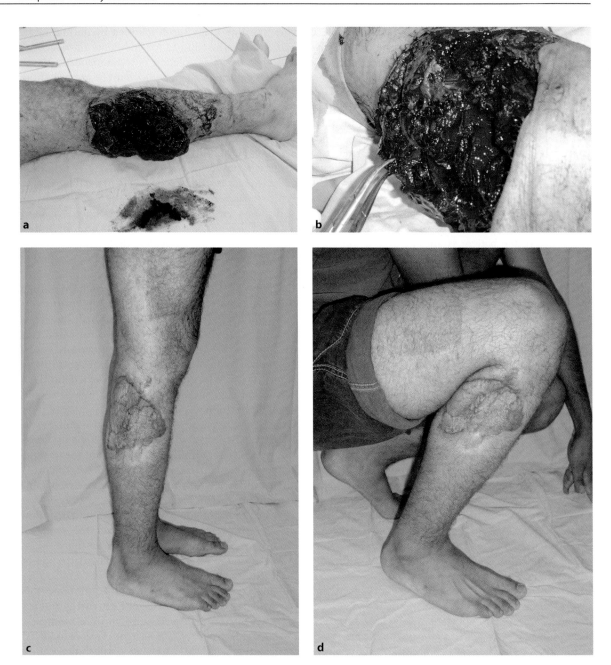

Fig. 2.2.1a–f. A 19-year-old male. Injury secondary to mine explosion affecting the right tibia. **a** Large crush wound on lateral aspect of proximal leg (before debridement). **b** Primary debridement with excision of necrotic and non-bleeding tissue was performed. Anatomical intact deep peroneal nerve was found. **c–f** Clinical pictures at the 12-months follow-up demonstrate wound healing with full range of movement of the ankle joint *(continues on next page)*

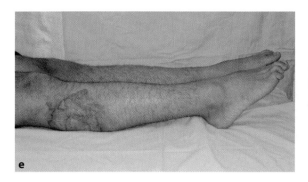
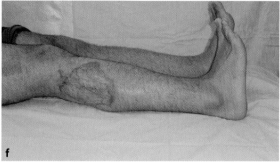

Fig. 2.2.1a–f. *(continued)* **c–f** Clinical pictures at the 12-months follow-up demonstrate wound healing with full range of movement of the ankle joint

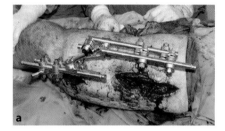
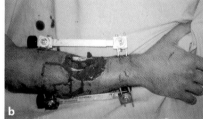

Fig. 2.2.2a,b. Clinical pictures of patients suffering from open high-energy limb fractures. An emergency procedure is carried out with stabilization of fractures with tubular AO (**a**) and Wagner (**b**) external fixators. The wounds are left open

ration and avoiding multiple surgical procedures in the future (Fig. 2.2.2).

For patients with vascular injuries (Gustilo IIIC fractures) or when open crush injury is significant, prophylactic fasciotomies must be performed. Compartment syndrome may occur in massively traumatized limbs and must be considered as a cause of limb ischemia. Swelling of muscle fibers to as much as 5 times normal size can be observed, and local edema may lead to compartment syndrome with further increase to the soft-tissue insult [35]. An open fracture does not automatically relieve the compartment of the injured limb, and even these patients can go on to develop compartment syndrome. Fasciotomy must be performed if any question of compartment syndrome exists. According to Moed and Fakhouri [96], prophylactic fasciotomy is indicated if there is the slightest indication that compartment syndrome will occur (Fig. 2.2.3).

If the wound is heavily contaminated and the soft-tissue damage is extensive, it is difficult to judge the extent of tissue excision. When finishing primary debridement procedures in patients suffering from high-energy injuries, primary closure of wounds must be avoided because of the contamination and retention of necrotic tissues. The widely accepted standard of care of soft-tissue injuries associated with open fractures is to leave the traumatic wound open after the initial surgical debridement [141].

During primary inspection and debridement of the wound, it is usually not possible to precisely assess the level and extent of the tissue damage and, as a general rule, meticulous repeated surgical debridements are required to achieve the best possible infection control. Repeated serial debridements are required for patients with high-velocity war injuries, especially those suffering from blast and crush injuries. A second-look procedure and repeated surgical debridement is to be performed under general anesthesia at 36- to 48-h intervals. This serial inspection under anesthesia and debridement of necrotic tissue should be undertaken until final closure is deemed to be safe (Fig. 2.2.4).

2.3 Vascular Injuries

Injuries with concomitant damage to the major extremity vessels require special consideration. Fox et al. [38] reported a high percentage of vascular injuries to the extremities in battle trauma. Life-threatening traumas to the head, chest, abdomen, and pelvis deserve priority, but delay in dealing with limb vessel trauma may be reflected in an adverse outcome. A high degree of

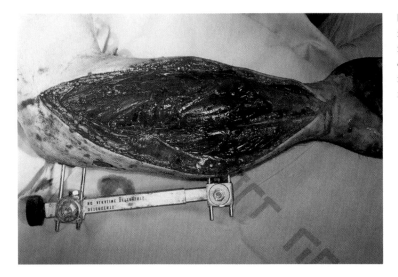

Fig. 2.2.3. A 33-year-old male with crush injury to the left forearm. Immediate fasciotomy was performed to handle acute compartment syndrome. The ulnar bone fracture is stabilized using a Wagner external fixation frame

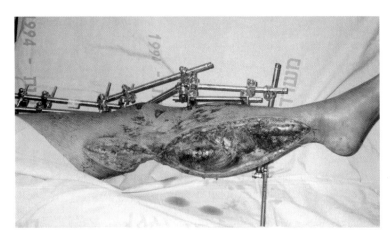

Fig. 2.2.4. Third day after severe motorcycle injury. Poor local condition with necrotic tissues dictates repeated surgical debridement

suspicion of vascular injury in high-energy trauma is mandatory, especially in peri-articular knee and elbow localizations, when treating fractures with gross displacement, and in patients with primary neurological deficits. Indications for immediate vascular surgery in such conditions are usually determined by a physical examination with special attention to pain, bleeding, pulsating masses, expanding hematomas, color of distal part of the extremity, paresthesia (or anesthesia), paralysis, and capillary refill time (signs of acute ischemia). A Doppler scan can be performed immediately in the emergency room or operating theatre. Angiographies or computer tomography are not usually useful in patients suffering from massive bleeding, and/or in a severe general condition, or in mass casualty situations [98]. Preoperative angiography and a CT-angio examination can be useful tools in patients in stable general and local conditions and when there is a high suspicion

of vascular injury to the limb, providing they do not endanger the limb by extending the ischemia time beyond permissible limits (Fig. 2.3.1).

Vascular repair must be performed as soon as possible. Surgical reconstruction in the "golden interval" – up to 4 h after injury – provides better functional results. The possibility of simultaneous damage to different vessels and damage to the same vessel at different anatomical levels must be suspected in the treatment of patients suffering from blast or shrapnel injuries. The ends of the injured vessels must be debrided and anastomosed. If an end-to-end suture is not possible, a reversed autogenous saphenous vein graft is the best alternative [95, 129]. According to Fox et al. [38], management of arterial repair with autologous vein graft remains the treatment of choice.

Immediate stable osteosynthesis is necessary to prevent thrombosis and occlusion, secondary damage

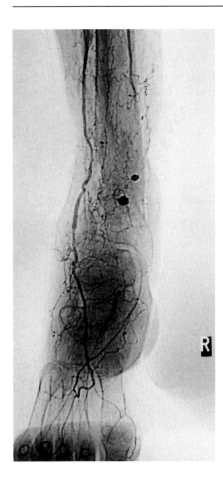

Fig. 2.3.1. Angiography of the right leg in a patient suffering from blast injury demonstrates occlusion of the anterior tibialis artery. Note radiological signs of foreign bodies above projection of ankle joint

treatment of patients suffering from blast or crush injuries with extensive tissue damage.

When more than 4 h has passed and limb ischemia is present, vascular reconstruction has priority over skeletal immobilization [98]. The time from injury to reperfusion can be shortened using a temporary intraluminal vascular bypass shunt, connected to both ends of the artery to reestablish arterial flow; establishment of blood flow to the distal extremity is achieved prior to stabilization. A simple unilateral external fixation frame must be applied, providing prompt fracture stabilization to protect the site of the vascular repair and offering adequate access to the wound for debridement and subsequent soft-tissue surgery, including final vascular reconstruction. This provides the vascular surgeon with a stable operative field. In addition, the temporary vascular shunt will facilitate the manipulation of the bone fragments in performing reduction and surgical stabilization. Now, having achieved a condition of bone stabilization, it is possible to perform definitive vascular reconstruction (Fig. 2.3.2).

The possibility of thrombosis of the repaired vessel dictates the desirability of surgical reconstruction of all the main injured vessels, if possible, in patients with multiple vascular damage in any limb segment (Fig. 2.3.3).

Prophylactic fasciotomy is necessary in reperfusion after vascular damage, compartment syndrome or distal limb ischemia. The leg is the most common site for the development of compartment syndrome of the lower limbs. The standard two-incision medial and lateral approach is by far the simplest and most effective method for decompressing all four compartments (Fig. 2.3.4, Fig. 2.3.5).

2.4 Peripheral Nerve Injury

According to Hopkinson and Marshall [56], small blood vessels are prone to rupture, while larger arteries are relatively resistant to injury (unless directly struck). Similarly, large nerve trunks are also rarely completely disrupted, while being susceptible to neurapraxia [57]. Most peripheral neurological injuries are neurapraxic and spontaneous recovery occurs frequently without exploration or repair of the nerve [13, 66]. According to Karas et al. [60], the majority of the nerve injuries sustained during gunshot wounds to the upper extremity are traction injuries. In unconscious or drugged patients and in patients with tourniquets, neurological diagnosis on admission may be very difficult. As soon as the casualty is able to cooperate, a rapid neurological examination must be done and recorded, starting at the medical aid station echelon [107]. The examination consists of asking the patent to gently move the limbs at all joints in all directions, as much as the wounds allow, and rapidly checking the limbs for loss of light touch.

to vascular anastomoses, and bleeding after vascular reconstruction. In the treatment of fractures with concomitant vascular injuries within the 4-h ischemia limit, we use the following surgical tactics:

- copious lavage of the wound and initial debridement;
- skeletal stabilization of the fracture using simple unilateral external fixation frame (assembly takes usually 20–30 min);
- further debridement;
- vascular reconstruction.

Thereby, we provide the necessary conditions for vascular repair: stability during vascular surgery and prevention of further damage to repaired vessels. Moreover, it is possible to fix the injured segment of the limb with shortening or angulation, releasing the site of the vascular repair from tension forces, especially in the

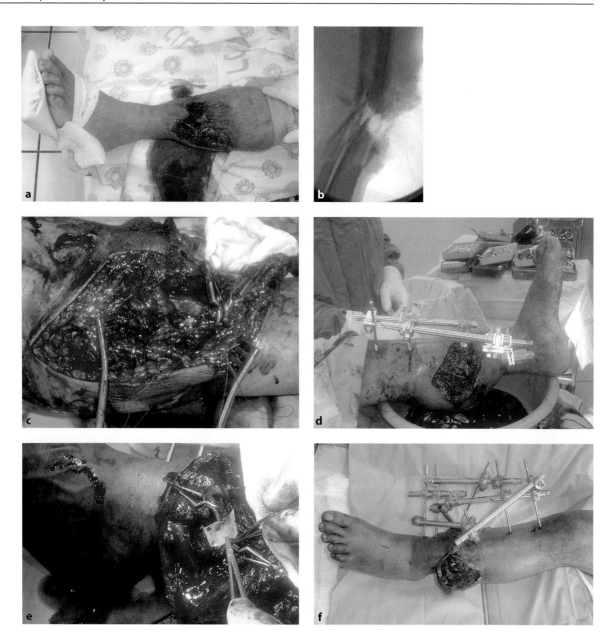

Fig. 2.3.2a–f. A 26-year-old male. Open Gustilo–Anderson type 3C tibial fracture with bone and soft-tissue loss secondary to blast injury. **a** Clinical picture on admission (6 h after injury). **b** Radiograph on admission demonstrates a comminuted fracture of tibial and fibular bones with bone loss. **c** Distal limb perfusion is restored using temporary intraluminal vascular bypass shunt to the tibialis anterior artery. **d** Primary stabilization of the tibial fracture with tubular external fixator is performed with shortening. **e** Clinical picture performed during final vascular reconstruction by end-to-end suture. **f** Final augmentation of the tubular external fixation frame is performed

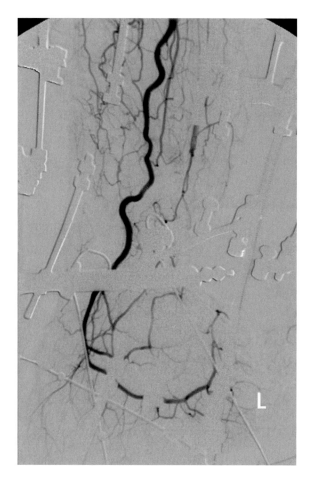

Fig. 2.3.3. Angiography performed on the third day after primary vascular reconstruction of anterior and posterior tibial arteries demonstrates thrombosis of anterior tibial artery

These findings should be interpreted in the light of knowledge of peripheral nerve anatomy and the site of penetrating or closed injuries. Electrodiagnostic studies are usually not helpful on admission and in the early post-injury period in seeking neural injuries, because they cannot distinguish between a neurapraxis lesion and a more serious injury [5]. Dynamic splints must be used in treating patients with post-traumatic peripheral nerve injuries since, in the early stage of management, avoiding pressure over anesthetic or hypoesthetic areas must be the rule. Daily gentle passive movements can help in preventing joint stiffness. Accordingly to Omer [103], 70% recovery of patients with peripheral nerve gunshot injuries to the upper extremities was observed, the majority of gains occurring over 3–6 months (average, 3–9 months). Brien et al. [13] reported that 60% of patients with peripheral nerve gunshot injuries to the lower extremities (sciatic and peroneal nerve) regained some degree of nerve function. According to Deitch and Grimes [26], the potential for long-term nerve in-

jury is highest in patients with high-velocity injuries and blasts, and they are also more often complicated by chronic pain and reflex sympathetic dystrophy. In 2003, Bartlett [4] concluded that acute repair seems to be rarely indicated for isolated gunshot nerve injuries to the extremities. When debriding a severe wound in the vicinity of a major nerve whose function is in doubt, the nerve should be explored without causing more soft-tissue damage in both proximal and distal directions from the contused area, until the appearance of the nerve is normal. Conditions are usually not good for primary or delayed primary nerve repair [107]. Nerve exploration is indicated, if a vascular injury is to be explored, after a negative change in neurological status after closed reduction and no clinically or electromyographically documented nerve function 3–6 months after injury [113, 145], or when a neurotmesis was observed and marked during wound debridement.

2.5 Primary Skeletal Stabilization

Unilateral external fixation quickly became established as a rapid, efficient, and relatively simple method of fracture stabilization, permitting vascular repair and control of the wound, retaining the distance between bone fragments and preventing contracture of the muscles, allowing mobilization of the limbs and facilitating evacuation, all of which are considerable advantages in the acute trauma setting [68]. The ease of mounting the unilateral external fixator is also a great advantage. Thus, we usually prefer unilateral external fixation frames for primary fracture stabilization.

After finishing the primary debridement procedure, all surgical instruments used for excision, drapes, and surgical gloves must be changed. The injured limb must be re-prepared and re-draped. The whole operated limb must be draped free: first, there must be continuous visual control of the color of the distal parts of the injured limb (including fingers or toes), capillary filling, and the possibility to palpate the peripheral arterial pulses. Second, severe and unusual trauma situations may dictate unorthodox approaches for the insertion of fixation elements from any direction. Third, adjoining joints must be seen during surgery to avoid unsuspected malpositioning (usually malrotation) of the bone fragments during the fixation procedure. Fourth, the possibility of extending an external fixation frame across adjoining joints with necessary temporary trans-articular bridging dictates a need to keep the operated limb fully exposed in these complex surgical situations (Fig. 2.5.1).

Prior to a half-pin insertion procedure, major vessels, nerves, musculo-tendinous units, large bone fragments, and pertinent skeletal landmarks should be marked on the skin. *The non-anatomical localization of important structures due to severe displacement of bone ends must be kept in mind!*

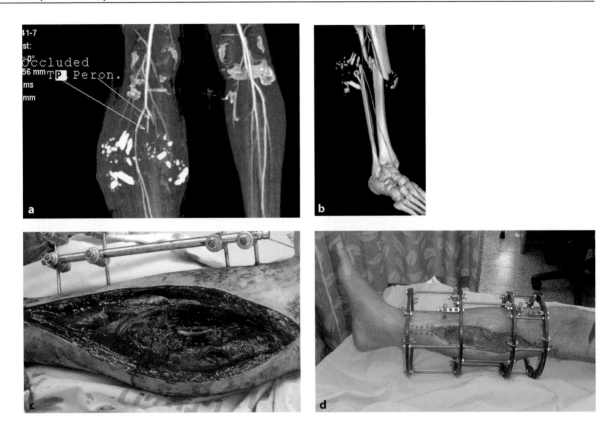

Fig. 2.3.4a–d. A 20-year-old male. Open Gustilo–Anderson type 3C tibial fracture secondary to anti-tank rocket blast injury. **a,b** CT-angio examination on admission demonstrates damage of posterior tibial and peroneal arteries of the right leg. **c** Primary debridement, fasciotomy, stabilization with tubular external fixator, and reconstruction of the posterior tibial artery and vein using a venous autograft was performed immediately. Clinical photo before partial closure of the wound for coverage of the vascular anastomoses site. **d** Follow-up 2 months after injury. Clinical photo demonstrates closure of soft-tissue defect by skin graft. Fixation of the tibial fracture by circular Ilizarov device

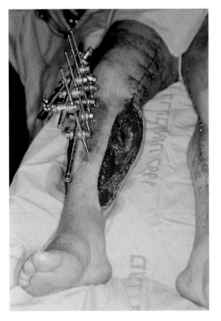

Fig. 2.3.5. A 23-year old male. Open Gustilo–Anderson type IIIC distal femoral fracture secondary to grenade blast injury. Primary debridement, fasciotomy, partial closure of exposed fracture site, and trans-knee stabilization with tubular external fixator were performed immediately

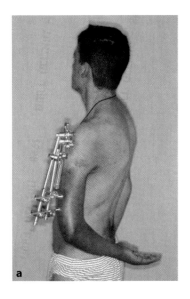

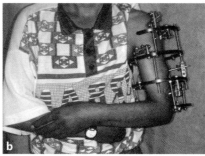

Fig. 2.5.1a,b. a Clinical appearance of intra-operatively missed malrotation of the humeral bone resulting from primary external fixation for an open humeral shaft fracture in a multi-injured patient. Orientation by means of the radiological image alone, but not by observing the clinical rotational malalignment, was the cause of this mistake. Note extensive internal malrotation of the upper limb. b This malrotation was repaired in a closed manner 3 weeks later, with conversion of the unilateral external fixator to the Ilizarov circular fixation frame

Unilateral tubular external fixation frames are usually used for primary fixation of bone fragments in treating patients with severe complex high-energy fractures with gross contamination. Unilateral external fixation devices with half-pins have a number of substantial advantages in the treatment of acute trauma, such as relative simplicity in assembling the frames and fixing the fracture, and have quickly established themselves as a quicker and easier method of primary fracture treatment than other methods of external fixation, especially in treating poly-traumatized patients. In our experience and in the current literature, the average time required to place a tubular external fixator is 20–30 min [68, 122]. This is a very important factor in the management of poly-traumatized patients and in mass casualty conditions. This frame configuration is stiff enough to maintain alignment under adverse loading situations, and is modular and sufficient for a wide variety of injuries. The unilateral configuration of the fixation device and the one-site technique for insertion of half-pins to the bone minimize the risk of iatrogenic soft-tissue damage, possible injury to the main vessels and nerves, and "trans-fixation" of the musculo-tendinous units, especially in treating proximal femoral and humeral bone fractures. The assembled unilateral fixation device allows the performing of initial debridement and secondary procedures on the soft tissues without removing the fixation frame. Many different external fixation systems for almost every bone in the body have been developed: AO, Hoffmann, Orthofix, Dinafix, EBI-fixators, etc. *Generally, use any type of frame you are trained to use, providing that it is quick and simple to apply.*

Our fixator of choice for primary stabilization is the AO (Synthes AG, Chur, Switzerland) tubular external fixator in a one-plane unilateral configuration. It is very simple and easy to learn, practical to use, and stiff and modular enough to accommodate a wide variety of situations [6]. A minimal number of different parts of the set allows a wide variety of frame assemblies. Usually, a pair of 5- to 6-mm threaded half-pins is introduced to both main bone fragments (proximal and distal). We prefer 6-mm half-pins due to greater bending stiffness and accordingly greater stability of the fracture fixation. For most femoral fractures, the half-pins are positioned at the lateral thigh, but for tibial fractures they may be placed either anteromedially or anterolaterally. To minimize post-fixation restriction of motion in adjacent joints, the half-pins must be inserted into the bone in functionally neutral zones and also in places with the least soft-tissue thickness. Each patient, especially after high-energy trauma with severe soft-tissue damage, needs an individual approach in choosing the right place for insertion of the half-pins. The better the condition of the skin and soft tissues at the insertion site, the less the possibility of developing local pin-related complications during the treatment period. If necessary, and if other appropriate sites for the insertion are absent, emergency temporary fracture stabilization can be performed by introducing the Schanz screw even to the uncovered bone. As soon as possible thereafter, this site must be covered by a soft-tissue flap, or the Schanz screw must be changed to another in a more acceptable location. The half-pin location must be planned to avoid disturbance of the nearby soft-tissue reconstructive procedures. A Kirschner wire, used as a probe, can help to determine the position of displaced bone fragments and to find the right sites for screw insertion. The widely recommended technique of low-speed and fractional drilling for half-pin insertion into the bone must be followed to avoid thermal damage to the hard and soft tissues. In addition, after performing an approximately 1-cm longitudinal skin incision, a triple trocar, including drill sleeve, must be used for bone drilling and also for introducing the half-pin to the bone to protect the surrounding soft tissues from thermal damage and from becoming twisted around the revolving instruments. The trocar must be centered on the bone before the drilling procedure. We recommend pre-drilling in the near and far cortex, because self-drilling half-pins, especially in the hands of insufficiently trained surgeons with relatively limited practical experience, can be dangerous for the surrounding soft tissues. The Schanz screws must be inserted across both cortices. Insertion of conical 6-mm half-pins into the bone must be accompanied by radiological control, because attempting to pull back a half-pin inserted too deeply results in significant diminution of the steadiness of the half-pin in the bone. The use of multi-directional half-pins can significantly increase the stability of the frame (Fig. 2.5.2).

A wide base of fixation (long lever arm) on each of the main bone fragments is desirable for improving stability of fixation. Insertion of half-pins into bone fragments close to the fracture zone must be performed at a distance of 4–5 cm from the ends of the bone fragments. The most proximal and distal half-pins are introduced into the bone near the metaphyseal zone (Fig. 2.5.3).

The wider the base of the external fixation frame, the more stable the fixation, the less the danger of pin loosening and local pin-tract infection, and the less the loss of reduction of the bone fragments. In addition, the wide base of the bone fragment fixation facilitates the management of bone fragments during the fracture reduction procedure. When dealing with short distal or proximal tibial or distal femoral fragments, it is desirable to fix with three half-pins, with two of them inserted into the metaphyseal zone at the same level (Delta frame). *Keep in mind localization of musculotendinous units and collateral ligaments to preserve the range of early post-operative motions* (Fig. 2.5.4).

Increasing the diameter of the half-pins and their number in each of the fragments of fixed bone greatly helps fixation stability. In treating large and obese patients with oblique fractures or severely comminuted bones and for the stabilization of femoral bone fractures, it is desirable to introduce three half-pins into the proximal and distal main fragments. Initially, the outer ends of the Schanz screws in each main bony fragment are connected by two short longitudinal tubes. Each of these proximal and distal blocks is then connected using tube–tube clamps to two intermediate connecting tubes. Manual reduction is stabilized by tightening tube-tube clamps on to connecting tubes. *Keep the rotational alignment in mind!* Reducing the distance between the bone and the longitudinal tube is important for increasing the stiffness of the frame. In peri-articular and intra-articular fractures, osteo-ligamentous injuries, severe intra-articular penetrating injuries, and damage to the capsule and ligamentary complex of joints adjoining the fracture site, there is a need for temporary trans-articular bridging of the injured limbs. In addition, this fixation is an effective tool for increasing stability in patients with fractures with a very short para-articular fragment. Technically, such fixation can be achieved by inserting two or three additional half-pins to the bony diaphysis from the opposite side of the fixed joint. The external ends of these half-pins are fixed to each other and then to the primary external fixation device, thereby stabilizing the fracture. Two tubes are enough for such a trans-articular crossing. Such a construction, although appearing outwardly to be massive, has relatively little weight and allows early patient mobilization, significantly easing nursing problems (Fig. 2.5.5, Fig. 2.5.6).

For the management of complex fractures of the upper limbs and performing primary surgical fixation of the relatively small forearm and hand bones, the use of small external fixators with 2.7- and 3.5-mm special Schanz screws is indicated. The rules and principles for using small external fixators are the same as for standard external fixation frames, including Delta configurations for temporary trans-articular bridging. These small external fixator configurations may be applied also to stabilize the small bones of the feet in treating complex trauma to the lower limbs. Additional percutaneous thin wire fixation may be required to optimize alignment and effect bone stabilization [55] (Fig. 2.5.7, Fig. 2.5.8).

Elimination of bone fragment displacement and anatomical reduction of the fractures at the stage of primary surgical debridement prevent pressure on the soft tissues and help uncomplicated wound healing. The fracture reduction procedure, performed in the acute phase of treatment, presents no significant technical difficulties, especially in open wound conditions in which the fracture zone and the bone fragments are exposed, resulting in a technically relatively easy open fracture reduction under vision. There is no significant resistance of the damaged soft tissues when performing the operative procedure in the acute period, because of the temporary post-traumatic paralysis of the muscles of the limb segment, which frequently exists. Furthermore, there is no stiffness in the neighboring joints. Thus it is desirable and possible even in the early stage of treatment to achieve the most precise anatomical reduction of the bone fragments. Great care must be taken to secure proper rotational alignment of the bone fragments before tightening the clamps. Accurate positioning of the bone fragments in the primary fixation frame is desirable, especially when taking into account that conversion to the final skeletal fixation may be delayed or even impossible in some patients due to a complex general

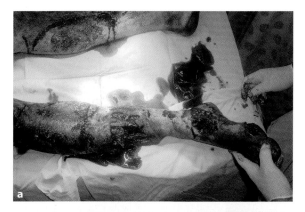

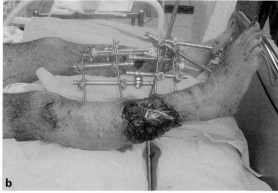

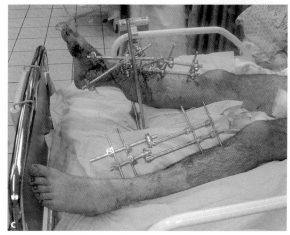

Fig. 2.5.2a–c. A 21-year-old soldier was injured by anti-tank rocket blast. **a** The clinical picture on admission demonstrates extensive lower limbs injury with massive tissue damage and loss. **b,c** Thorough debridement was performed. The fractures of both legs are aligned and stabilized using AO tubular external fixation frames. Clinical right- and left-side views of the lower limbs after primary fixation. Note trans-ankle bridging on the right lower limb

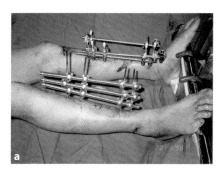

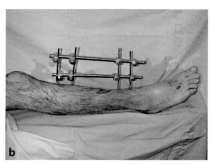

Fig. 2.5.3a,b. Clinical appearance of stabilization of tibial fractures by unilateral AO external fixation frames

condition [51]. However, precise anatomical reduction of the bone fragments at the stage of performing primary wound debridement in patients with high-energy injuries cannot be an end in itself, especially in a grave general condition or multiply injured patients. *It is important that over-distraction, used primarily for reduction of bone fragments, is released during final stabilization of the external fixator.* (Fig. 2.5.9)

The surgical procedure for treating these patients must be minimally traumatic and performed as soon as possible, so as to be least disruptive of the patient's general condition and the local tissue status. The aim is to achieve stable fixation by eliminating gross bone fragment displacement and to relieve pressure on the skin and neuro-vascular structures. However, the quality and radicality of the primary surgical debridement must be preserved, as together they determine the prognosis of uncomplicated wound healing. The extensive possibilities of the Ilizarov method in tissue genesis provide an answer for almost any type of bone damage,

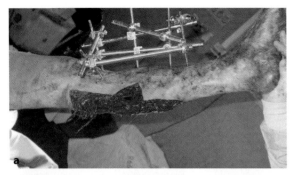

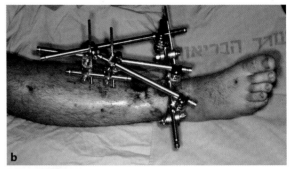

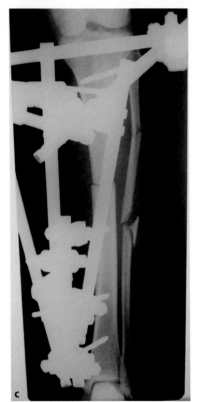

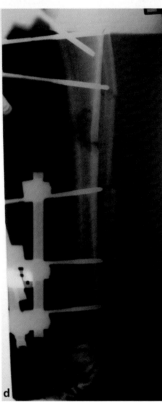

Fig. 2.5.4a–d. Clinical (**a,b**) and radiological (**c,d**) views of Delta frames mounting for external skeletal stabilization

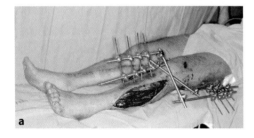

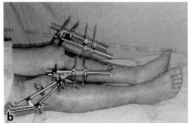

Fig. 2.5.5a,b. Temporary trans-knee bridging using AO tubular external fixation frames

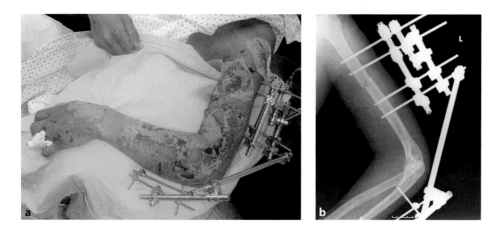

Fig. 2.5.6a,b. Temporary trans-elbow bridging using AO tubular external fixation frame

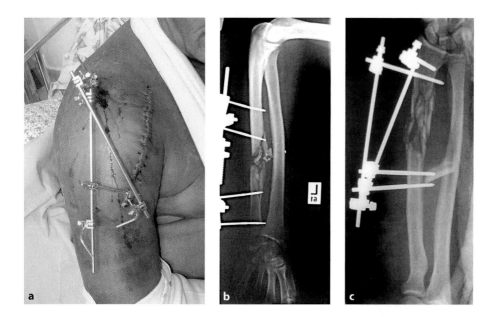

Fig. 2.5.7a–c. Stabilization of **a** humeral, **b** ulnar, and **c** and radial fractures using small external fixation sets

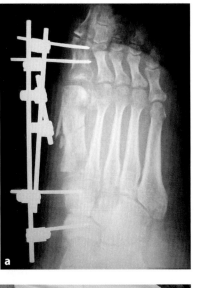

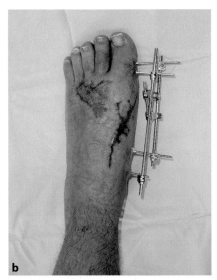

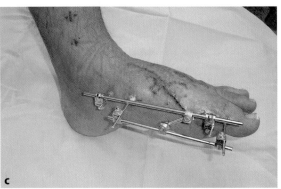

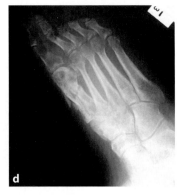

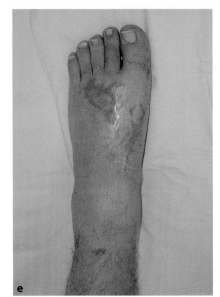

Fig. 2.5.8a–g. A 20-year-old male. This victim of a motorcycle accident sustained a crush injury to his left foot with open comminuted fractures of the first ray. Mini-external fixation frames maintain stabilization. **a** Postoperative radiological pictures. **b,c** Clinical appearance 4 weeks after injury. **d,e** The external fixation frame was removed 2 months after the trauma. Clinical and radiological appearance after fixator removal. **f,g** *see next page*

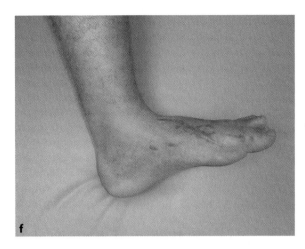
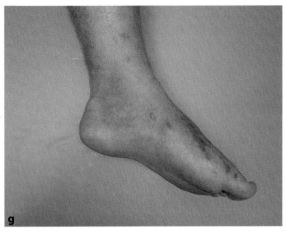

Fig. 2.5.8a–g. *(continued)* **f,g** The external fixation frame was removed 2 months after the trauma. Clinical and radiological appearance after fixator removal

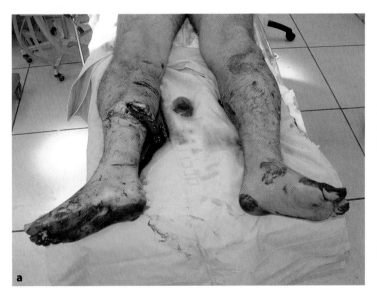
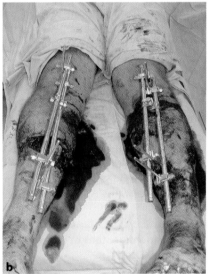

Fig. 2.5.9a,b. a Clinical picture of the lower limbs in a multi-injured patient in critical general condition. **b** Note that only axial re-alignment and external fixation were performed on admission for the high-energy compound tibial fractures for emergency stabilization

including massive bone loss. In our opinion, the condition of the soft tissues, especially the severity and extent of the primary damage and loss, is the main determining factor in both the treatment and prognosis of high-energy injuries.

2.6 Soft-Tissue Protection by External Fixation Frames

Prolonged immobilization, particularly in trans-articular fixation, results in constant pressure on the skin and soft tissues of the posterior aspect of the limbs in supine patients and may be a complicating factor, especially involving the heels of unconscious patients or those with denervation of the limbs. We add elements in assembling the external fixator to achieve limb suspension and prevent compression of the posterior compartment caused by the weight of the limb and the external fixator [72]. This can be done by positioning a portion of the standard tubing across the mattress with two other tube sections obliquely attached so as to form a triangular assembly (apex at the anterior fixation rod, base across the mattress) through which the patient's limb projects. A similar modification can be used with a large ring from a circular Ilizarov frame which is easily attached to the half-pin of the unilateral external fixator. An additional important benefit is that the posterior aspect of the limb is exposed for any necessary treatment, including operative procedures (Fig. 2.6.1).

An external fixation frame extension for limb suspension can alleviate constant pressure on the soft tissues and prevent pressure sores in patients with altered consciousness (head injuries, sedation, and sensory deficit) [118]. Furthermore, this simple attachment, holding the limb segment in the necessary position, can be used to facilitate operative procedures (Fig. 2.6.2, Fig. 2.6.3).

2.7 The Management of Retained Bullets in the Limbs

In high-energy injuries, retained missile fragments encountered during debridement are removed during the procedure. Removing these fragments from the wound cavity causes little additional trauma and can significantly lower the potential for sepsis [127]. A thorough search should be made to remove not only radiographically detected metal fragments, but also other incidental debris, including fragments of clothing, skin, and hair. In our experience in treating mine blast victims, we often found fragments of stones during surgical debridement.

The need to remove the foreign bodies depends primarily on the location of the retained missile [18]. Missiles retained in the joints or bursa can result in mechanical abrasion, mechanical obstruction and destructive arthritis, leading to arthropathy and systemic lead toxicity of the central nervous system, the peripheral nervous system, and the gastrointestinal, renal, and hematological systems, and, therefore, missiles should be removed, arthroscopically if possible. Arthrotomy is often necessary for adequate debridement, followed by surgical restoration of the articular surface but, in uncomplicated cases, arthroscopy can provide valuable diagnostic information and definitive treatment [106]. In addition to avoiding the morbidity associated with arthrotomy, arthroscopy allows easier access to intra-articular areas which are difficult to visualize, such as the posterior aspects of the knee joint. The literature suggests that patients with retained intra-articular lead bullets after gunshot wounds are at risk for the development of systemic lead poisoning [28, 149]. Aggressive surgical therapy may be needed for these patients [131] (Fig. 2.7.1).

Removing the intra-articularly placed foreign bodies is best performed in the early stages of treatment but is not a life-saving procedure, especially in the management of multi-injured patients, and can be postponed if necessary. Open or arthroscopic removal of bullets or other foreign bodies is performed in these patients as an elective procedure [149]. Foreign bodies close to neurovascular formations and irritating them must be removed as soon as possible, taking great care (Fig. 2.7.2).

In later stages of treatment, there may be indications for removing foreign bodies that provoke septic complications. Foreign bodies that cause unpleasant and painful feelings upon movement, from wearing clothing and shoes, and foreign bodies that are easily palpated under the skin are usually removed at later stages. However, it is difficult, and sometimes impossible, to remove all missile fragments that are retained in the limbs. The morbidity of the removal procedure can be significant. Excellent long-term results can be achieved without the routine removal of missile fragments.

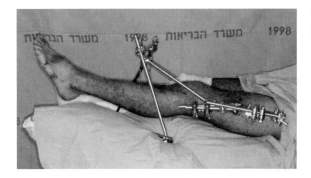

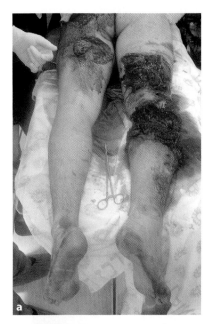

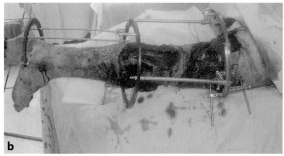

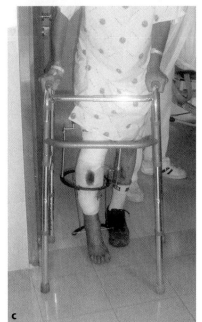

Fig. 2.6.1. External fixation frame extension for pressure sore prevention

Fig. 2.6.2a–e. A 21-year-old soldier sustained a right lower limb injury caused by the blast of an anti-tank rocket. Debridement of the wounds was performed immediately on admission. **a** Clinical photo at time of admission. **b** Clinical photo after surgical debridement and fixation of the injured lower limb in the large-size circular frame for protection of soft tissues. **c** Two weeks after injury – early walking with toe touch to the injured lower limb. **d,e** *see next page*

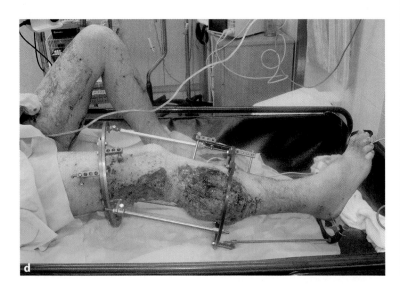

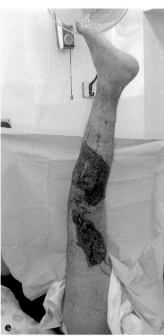

Fig. 2.6.2a–e. *(continued)* **d** Three weeks after injury. Ilizarov external fixator served as protection frame for injured limb. Clinical photo demonstrates good coverage of the wound surface by skin grafts. **e** Protective external frame was removed 4 weeks after injury. Clinical appearance of the lower limb at 2-month follow-up

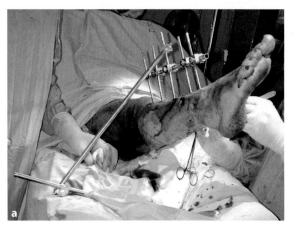

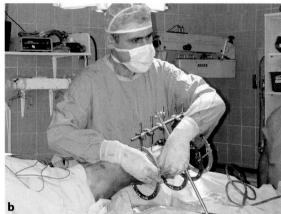

Fig. 2.6.3a,b. Extension of the external fixation frame to elevate the position of the injured limb during surgery can be a useful tool for more comfortable performance of the operative procedure

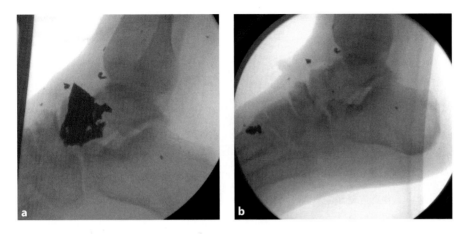

Fig. 2.7.1a,b. A 21-year-old soldier sustained a right lower limb injury caused by the blast of an anti-tank rocket. **a** Radiograph on admission shows a large foreign body in the subtalar joint. **b** The foreign body was removed during primary debridement on admission

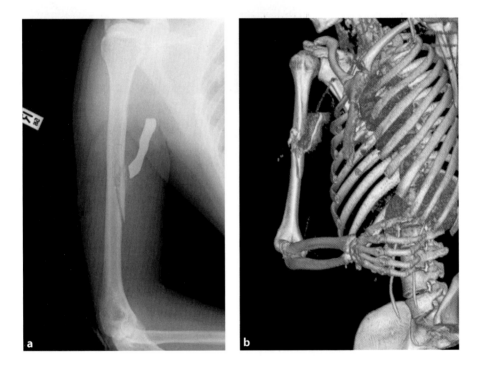

Fig. 2.7.2a–f. A 20-year-old soldier sustained a right proximal arm wound caused by anti-tank rocket. Debridement and exploration of the wound were performed immediately on admission. **a** Radiograph on admission shows fracture of the humeral bone by a large metal foreign body. **b** 3D CT-angio demonstrates damage to the brachial artery. **c–f** *see next page*

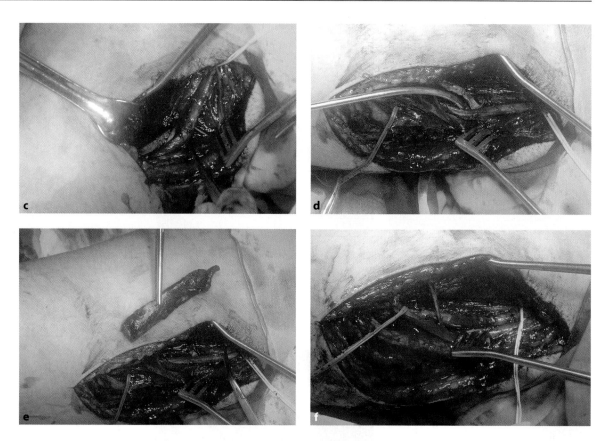

Fig. 2.7.2a–f. *(continued)* **c** Clinical photo at time of exploration. Note pressure on the neurovascular bundle by a large foreign body. **d** Removing the foreign body. **e** The large metal foreign body is removed. Note the vascular clamp on the proximal end of the injured brachial artery. **f** The brachial artery is reconstructed using autologous interpositional vein grafting

Definitive Reconstruction

3.1 Final Soft-Tissue Coverage

The fracture site and the bone fragments should ideally be covered with soft tissue to prevent bone desiccation and secondary necrosis and osteomyelitis. Stable immobilization of the fracture is an essential precondition for successful soft-tissue closure, providing optimal conditions for soft-tissue healing and averting further soft-tissue damage [128]. The final soft-tissue coverage can usually be performed 5–7 days after injury, depending on the mechanism of injury, wound status, general condition of the patient, and availability of appropriate expertise in orthopedic and plastic surgery. Surgical debridement also should be repeated at the time of the final soft-tissue reconstruction. The reconstruction of soft tissues is a difficult aspect of limb salvage after high-energy extremity injury. The reconstructive procedures for soft tissues are chosen according to the patient's general condition, wound location and extent of surface area cover lost, depth of tissue damage, and quality of surrounding tissues [138]. Traditionally, soft-tissue defects have been closed in a variety of ways. Small wounds may be allowed to heal secondarily. Delayed primary sutures are used mainly in patients in whom there is a clean wound with little soft-tissue damage, without significant tissue loss. It should be noted that the leg has minimal skin reserves so that even minor skin excision during debridement procedures may preclude skin edge approximation. This procedure is usually technically possible within the first 10 days after injury, when the skin edges are still mobile and may be approximated easily. Residual skin tension after placement of sutures must be avoided.

Skin grafting becomes preferable when tension is required for closure [5]. Skin grafts can be used only on muscle, fascia or fat tissue; they should be applied on well-vascularized granulation tissue. Split skin grafts cannot cover bone, tendon, open joint or fracture sites. Local and distant sliding tissue flaps and free tissue transfer may be employed for covering wounds in patients with tissue loss. Restoration of the well-vascularized soft-tissue envelope enhances vascularity at the fracture site, promotes fracture healing, allows delivery

of antibiotics, and prevents secondary wound contamination, desiccation, and damage to bone, articular cartilage, tendons, and nerves [146]. The flap should have adequate circulation and be larger than the primary defect.

The cross leg flap, where a large fasciocutaneous flap is elevated on one leg to cover a defect on the other, is very rarely used these days but may, on occasion, provide a useful salvage covering procedure when other options are either unavailable or have failed [67]. Tissue transfer in a stepwise fashion on a wrist carrier requires prolonged bizarre positioning of patients and is not used in the modern surgical practice for the treatment of trauma patients (Fig. 3.1.1).

Free microvascular tissue transfer is required for patients with extensive soft-tissue loss, where local options are limited [30, 67, 89, 116]. The advantage of the free tissue transfer is not only coverage of extensive soft-tissue defects, but also improved perfusion at the host site by muscle transplantation. The enhanced transport of oxygen-rich blood, together with some improvement in the body's intrinsic defenses against infection in the area of the lesion, will convert a "non-osteogenic" or "partially osteogenic" site into a "highly osteogenic" site [128]. According to Hammert et al. [49], the presence of highly vascularized soft tissue provides a local environment favorable for wound healing and earlier return to activities of life. Moreover, a bulky free vascular muscular graft can be a useful tool for handling dead space, especially when segmental bone loss has occurred. We prefer the technique of wound cover using a latissimus dorsi muscle flap with free microvascular tissue transfer. Free vascular muscular grafts will decrease the rate of wound complications and increase the rate of limb salvage.

Vacuum-assisted closure (VAC) (KCI, San Antonio, TX) is selected for patients in a poor general condition and for those who refuse a more complicated procedure. Exposed bone, single artery perfusion of the leg, and severe contusion of the surrounding tissue are also considered as indications for a VAC procedure. By performing continuous negative suction, progressive stretching of the surrounding tissue is achieved. It is believed that VAC devices produce arteriolar dilatation, decrease ex-

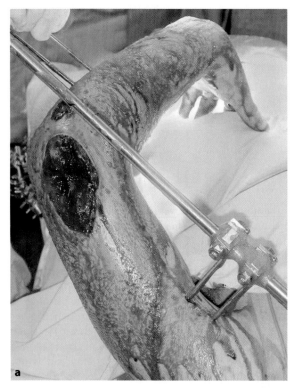

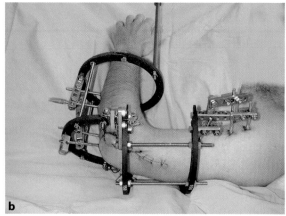

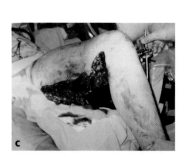

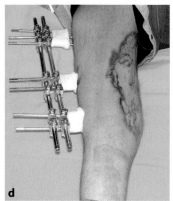

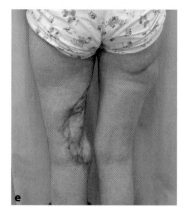

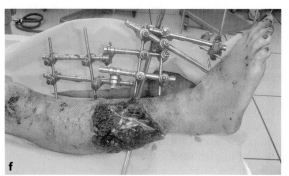

Fig. 3.1.1a–l. Final surgical coverage of wounds using: **a,b** delayed primary sutures; **c,d,e** skin grafts; **f** local fasciocutaneous flap; **g–l** *see next page*

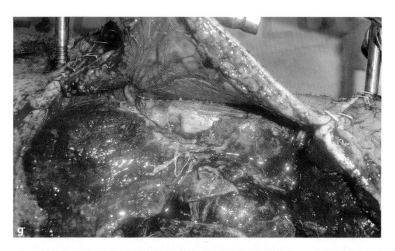

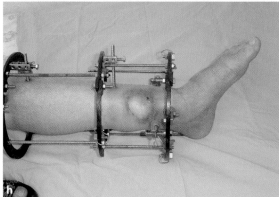

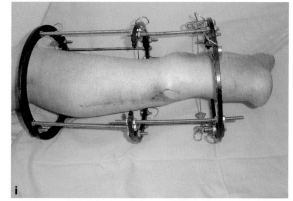

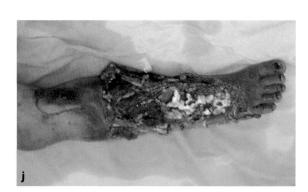

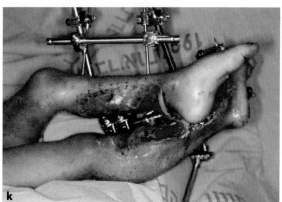

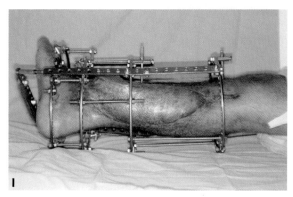

Fig. 3.1.1a–l. *(continued)* **g** local fasciocutaneous flap; **h,i** local skin-muscle tissue flap; **j,k** cross-leg fasciocutaneous flap; **l** free microvascular tissue transfer

cess fluid, improve microcirculation and eliminate cytokines, collagenases and other factors known to inhibit wound healing [54]. A decrease in the bacterial count has also been noted [97]. Vacuum-assisted closure has the advantage of producing granulating tissue over exposed tendons, bones or hardware, which can be skingrafted later [25] (Fig. 3.1.2).

The unique possibilities of guided graduated tissue translation and distraction in the external fixation frame can also be successfully used for elimination of soft-tissue defects in some patients. The Ilizarov device can be used for skin expansion to cover an exposed fracture or bone. To use this technique, a small reconstruction mandibular plate must be sutured to the skin edge of the wound and tied to the plate of the Ilizarov device. Incremental, daily, guided traction can be applied to the skin edge for gradual coverage of the exposed bone. After completing the coverage procedure and achieving skin edge contact, the skin edges can be sutured one to another without any skin grafting or free

tissue transfer. The use of this method is easily and reliably combined with the advantages of the Ilizarov device, yielding slowly expanded skin with a good blood supply for management of an open fracture with skin and soft-tissue defects, involving the anterior edge of the tibial shaft that is not "padded" with muscle tissue [75] (Fig. 3.1.3).

3.2 Definitive Skeletal Reconstruction

Exact fracture reduction and stable bone fixation should be performed after final coverage of the wounds has been achieved. However, unilateral external fixation, as a definitive method of skeletal stabilization in patients suffering from high-energy injuries, has been associated with a high rate of non-union [59, 85, 117]. Various methods of definitive fracture fixation have been used. Conversion of a temporary external fixation frame to internal fracture fixation, including meth-

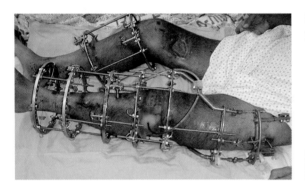

Fig. 3.1.2. Using vacuum-assisted closure for a severely injured patient with exposed fracture site

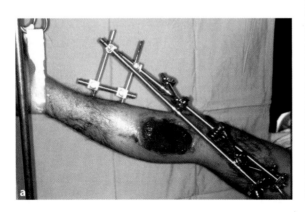

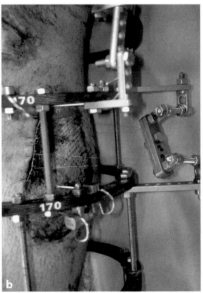

Fig. 3.1.3a–f. Skin expansion by Ilizarov device in treating a 21-year-old soldier who sustained a gunshot proximal tibial fracture with exposed bone and fracture site. **a** Clinical appearance of left lower limb on 3rd day after admission demonstrates unilateral trans-knee external fixation. Note open wound on the anterolateral surface of the leg with the exposed anterior edge of the tibial bone. **b** Mandibular Reconstruction Plate (Mathys Medical, Bettlach, Switzerland) is sutured to the wound edge and connected to the Ilizarov plate by stainless steel sutures. **c–f** *see next page*

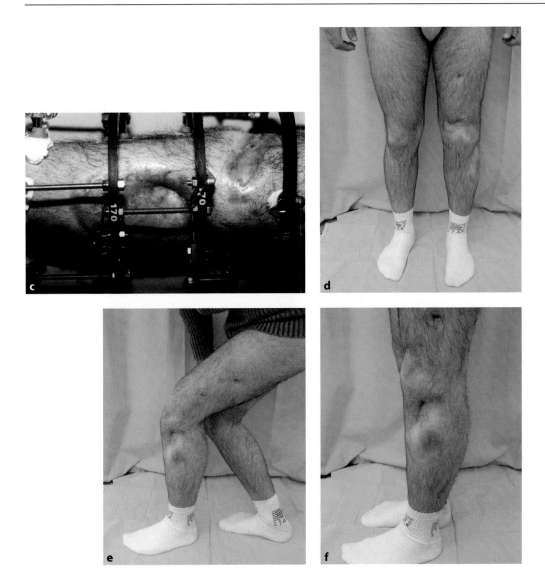

Fig. 3.1.3a–f. *(continued)* **c** The wound is closed after advancement of the stretched anterior edge of the wound. **d–f** One year after injury, the wound is closed and the patient is fully ambulatory. *Reproduced with permission from © Lippincott Williams and Wilkins; Lerner et al (2000) Using the Ilizarov external fixation device for skin expansion. Ann Plast Surg 45:535–537 [75]*

ods of intramedullary locking, nailing and plating, is a common and convenient method of definitive skeletal stabilization in patients with low-energy injuries. However, in the presence of severe and extensive soft-tissue injury in the fracture zone, any surgical approach for open reduction of displaced bone fragments and the introduction and fixing of a surgical implant will act as additional trauma to the soft tissues, with the attending possibilities of disturbing local circulation and vascularization of the fracture site. Furthermore, these patients usually have a problem with coverage of the fracture site and bone ends. Any method of internal fixation can be a relatively risky procedure, hazarding septic complications by the presence of a metal fixator as an additional massive foreign body. These problems are especially acute when treating victims of combat trauma and terror attacks, where multiple foreign bodies can be present in the fracture zone and surrounding soft tissues. Therefore, to prevent the development of dangerous complications, we recommend performing final fracture stabilization with a multi-dimensional and multi-functional method of definitive circular/hybrid external fixation [76].

The process of achieving good reduction in the final outcome must take into account the possibility of severe frequent complications of reduction surgery in the treatment of high-energy fractures. Contrary to internal fixation methods, it is not necessary to wait for final and safe fracture site coverage when using external fixation frames, and bone reconstructive procedures can be carried out in the early post-trauma period. This is a very important factor, because the possibilities for closed fracture reduction are diminished while waiting for the process of organization of the fracture hematoma (Fig. 3.2.1, Fig. 3.2.2, Fig. 3.2.3).

Skeletal fixation in treating multiply injured patients should commence with the segment which is non-displaced or minimally displaced. Then, proceed to the cross-over fixation of fractures with more significant displacement. The opposite sequence of actions, leaving non-displaced or minimally displaced fractures to the final stage of the operation and performing manipulations on the other limb's more displaced segments, creates the hazard of losing the acceptable fracture alignment of the initially undisplaced or least displaced bone fragments which were left unfixed at the beginning.

In the unilateral fixation frames, there is very limited potential for influence on the bone fragments during the fracture reduction procedure. In patients with an acceptable emergency reduction, fixation in a unilateral external fixation frame can be continued until bone healing is completed. However, in many patients, the primary tubular external fixation of the emergency condition has to be changed to a hybrid or ring system to achieve final reduction and stabilization of the fracture site. In order to perform this transition efficiently with minimal additional trauma to the patient, we use the half-pins from the primary tubular external fixator which were applied in the emergency treatment and add more tension wires and additional half-pins for stable reduction and final fixation of bone fragments. To preserve the primary alignment, redundant parts of the tubular external fixator are removed only after the final hybrid frame is built and the fracture fixed. In some cases, the technical assembly of the circular frame can be carried out outside the operating room, thereby shortening the operating time, as only additional tension wires and half-pins need to be inserted under anesthesia in the operating theatre (Fig. 3.2.4).

3.2.1 Ilizarov Circular Fixation

Five to seven days following trauma, or when the general and soft-tissue conditions permit, the unilateral tubular external fixator can be exchanged for a circular fixation frame that enables full weight-bearing (Fig. 3.2.1.1, Fig. 3.2.1.2).

Taking into consideration the availability of many publications dealing with the Ilizarov method and its application in various orthopedic and trauma conditions, we limit ourselves here to describing the fundamental principles that are required in the treatment of severe complex fractures of the limbs.

Additional fluoroscopy before the final reconstructive operation is useful for the diagnosis of missed fractures, foreign bodies, or for finding more distant extensions of the fracture.

During surgery to the thigh, the patient is placed in the supine position with a small sand-bag elevation under the buttocks or lumbar zone on the side of the injury. This prevents soft-tissue deformation of the thigh muscle and skin mass caused by the supine position and, as a result, prevents trans-fixation of the soft tissues by thin wires and half-pins in a non-anatomical shifted position upon fixation of the bone fragments. Non-compliance with these simple positioning principles results in excessive tension on the skin and soft tissues around the implanted wires and pins, with ensuing pain, pin-tract infection, and joint stiffness. Detecting such soft-tissue deformities in the final stage of the operation, it is necessary to release skin tension by small incisions of the skin over the corresponding wires and pins; for gross soft-tissue deformities and severe soft-tissue tension, it is better to re-insert the offending wire or Schanz screw. When performing surgery on the leg (calf), the elevation bolster is placed under the thigh, providing free muscle positioning on the posterior aspect of the calf, and avoiding flattening of the calf under its own weight.

To ensure sterile conditions, it is better to remove the primarily placed unilateral external fixation frame before preoperative cleaning. At this time, the tubes of the unilateral frame are removed and the stability of fixation

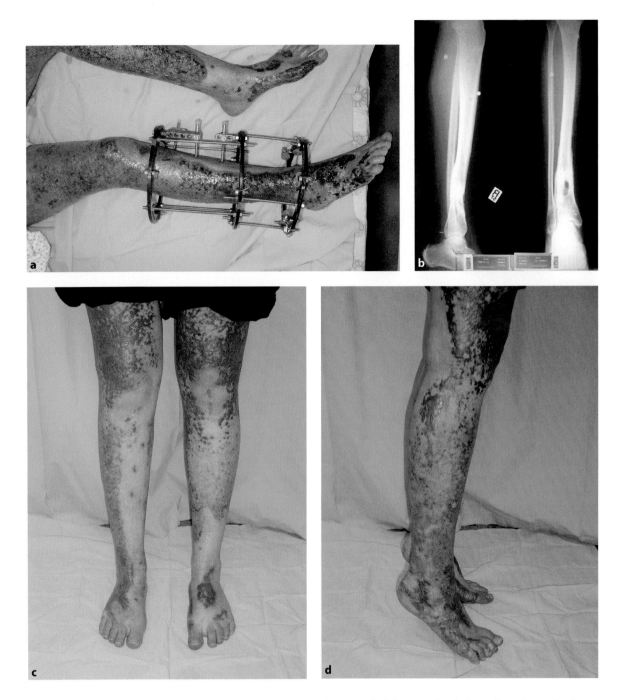

Fig. 3.2.1a–g. A 19-year-old female, after a bus blast injury. Complex open tibial fracture of right leg and circular grade 3 burns involving both legs. In this situation, we recommend a minimally invasive procedure with the use of the circular Ilizarov external fixation frame for fracture stabilization and skin graft protection. **a** Clinical appearance of the lower limbs 2 weeks after burn injury. Right tibial fracture is fixed by circular Ilizarov frame. **b** One-year follow-up. Radiological pictures of solid union of the fractures. **c–d** Clinical appearance demonstrates full range of movement of the knee and ankle joints at 1-year follow-up. **e–g** *see next page*

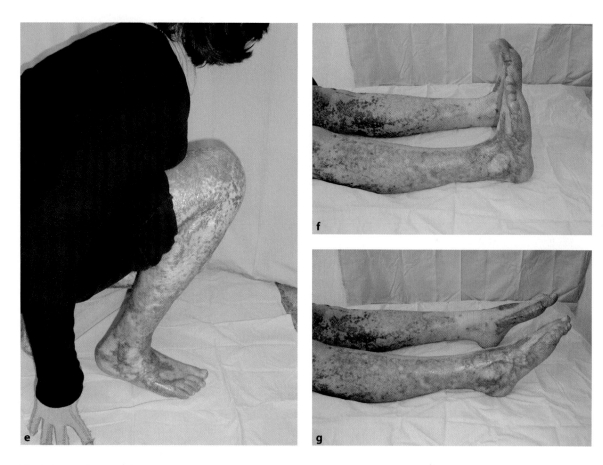

Fig. 3.2.1a–g. *(continued)* **e–g** Clinical appearance demonstrates full range of movement of the knee and ankle joints at 1-year follow-up

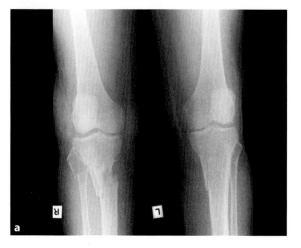

Fig. 3.2.2a–e. A 55-year-old male with bilateral proximal tibial fractures due to road traffic accident as a pedestrian. **a** Radiological appearance on admission. **b–e** *see next page*

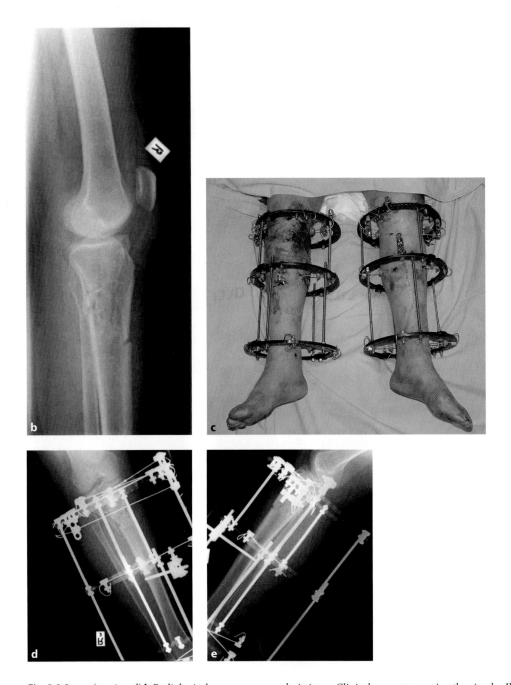

Fig. 3.2.2a–e. *(continued)* **b** Radiological appearance on admission. **c** Clinical appearance using the circular Ilizarov external fixation frames for bilateral fracture stabilization with the presence of blisters on the right leg. **d,e** Post-operative radiographs demonstrate stabilization of the fractures in position of reduction

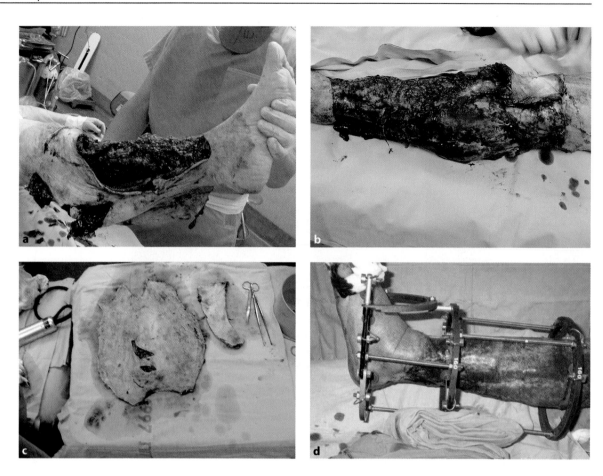

Fig. 3.2.3a–d. A 69-year-old female with crush injury to her right leg with degloving due to road traffic accident as a pedestrian. **a** Clinical photo on admission. Note the circular degloving of the leg. **b** Clinical photo of the leg after surgical debridement. **c** After excision of subcutaneous fat tissue, the degloved skin is ready for replantation. **d** Clinical view of the leg after skin replantation and Ilizarov trans-ankle external fixation

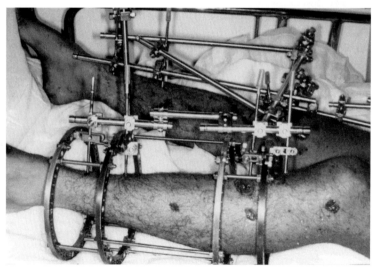

Fig. 3.2.4. Final circular frame (left leg) can be built outside the operating room on the basis of the unilateral tubular fixator with preservation of alignment. Additional tension wires need to be inserted under anesthesia in the operating theatre. *Lerner et al. Modular use of external fixation configurations for treatment of complex and severely injured limbs. Eur J Trauma 2003; 29:108–111 [77] (© Urban & Vogel. Reproduced with permission)*

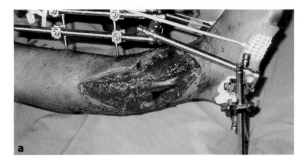
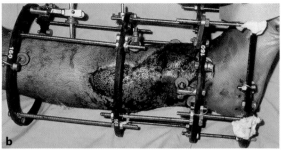

Fig. 3.2.1.1a,b. A 12-year-old male. This victim of a road mine blast injury sustained an open fracture of the right distal tibia and fibula. He was treated 3 h after the accident with surgical debridement and external fixation with a hybrid frame. **a** Clinical photo of the right leg 7 days after injury. The fractured bones stabilized using a hybrid external fixation frame. **b** Conversion of primary placed hybrid fixation frame to circular Ilizarov fixator and closure of soft-tissue wound using skin grafting were performed on the 7th day after trauma. Clinical appearance of the right lower limb 2 weeks after surgery

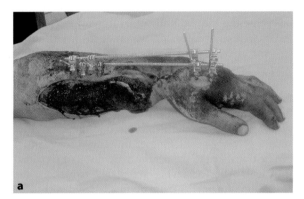
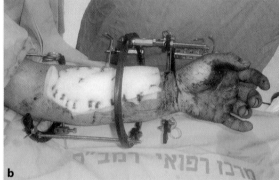

Fig. 3.2.1.2a,b. A 20-year-old male in a mine blast sustained an open fracture of the left distal radial bone. He was treated on admission with surgical debridement and external fixation using a Mini AO external fixation frame. **a** Clinical photo of the left forearm after primary stabilization of the fracture by mini AO external fixator. **b** Conversion of primary placed tubular fixation frame to circular Ilizarov fixator performed 5 days later; the skin defect was covered using skin graft

of each half-pin in the bone is examined. Unstable half-pins, half-pins with signs of local infection, and pins located over tendon-muscle units must be removed.

Various methods of frame assembly exist: preliminary mounting of the frame before surgery; mounting the circular frame around the fixed limb segment during surgery; and separate mounting of the proximal and distal fixation blocks set in a position of re-alignment and connected together after fixation to the corresponding main bone fragments. As a rule, high-energy injuries to the limbs result in utter instability of the injured limb. Early and reliable stabilization of the injured segment is necessary to prevent additional trauma to the soft tissues, and also for better anatomical orientation of the wound. For this reason, we recommend assembling the fixation circular frame before surgery. We prefer a diameter of rings that is at least 2–3 cm larger

than the maximal diameter of the operated limb segment. After fitting the frame on the injured segment of the limb and correcting the ring locations in the fixed bone segments, the frame is stabilized with the nuts. If stabilization of the frame is not executed at this early stage of the surgery, one or two loose nuts found later result in a loss of the entire system's stability, and also in a loss of the frame's reduction effectiveness. Moreover, the forces acting during the guided transfer of displaced bone fragments will result in unexpected deformities of the fixation frame itself. This mistake can cause technical difficulties and wastes considerable effort and time, necessitating a repetition of earlier stages of the operative procedure.

Performing stabilization of the tibial fracture, we start the procedure by inserting the proximal reference metaphyseal thin wire, which must be introduced from the anterolateral site of the shin (proximal or anterior to the fibular head), in a postero-medial direction in the plane of the articular surface of the knee. Low-speed drilling with frequent stops is used to insert a thin wire into the bone. Using his/her free hand and holding a pad moistened in alcohol for additional disinfection and cooling of the wire, the surgeon directs the thin wire. After puncturing the skin and soft tissue and impinging onto the bone, and before proceeding with the drilling, it is desirable to thrust and compress the soft tissues by hand onto the bone; this simple maneuver diminishes the tendency of the soft tissue to be caught up and twist around the rotating wire, creating additional soft-tissue damage.

The thin wire must be tensioned to 130 kg and fixed in the proximal ring of the fixation frame. Remember: when performing tightening of the wire to the ring, the head of the fixation bolt should be held stationary with one wrench while turning the nut with another. If the non-fixed bolt turns during the tightening procedure, the thin wire will bend, resulting in a change of tension. The assistant, holding the foot, performs manual axial distraction in the rotational alignment position (orientation of the foot and knee; the knee joint must remain uncovered throughout the surgery). The distal tibial bone fragment must be fixed in the distal ring of the frame using another reference wire inserted in the supramalleolar zone from the postero-medial site in the anterolateral direction. Insertion of both these wires must be guided by intraoperative radiography; parallel positioning according to the knee and ankle joint line is desirable. Insertion of the para-articular wires in a position deviating from the joint line can be a cause of mal-angulation of the main bone fragments after tensioning and fixation of the wires into the pre-assembled hard frame. A similar mal-angulation of the bone fragments can be observed also by performing fixing of inter-rings placed by threaded rods by assembly of the fixation frame on the limb during operation. A small deviation from parallel is not an indication for reinserting the wires; this can be corrected by adding washers or by fixing the wire ends to the opposite sides of the ring (according to the deviated wire's deflection). Sideways displacement of the bone fragments can result after tensioning of obliquely inserted proximal and distal para-articular wires.

The wire fixator must be aligned with the corresponding wire (but never bend the wire to fit the fixator), because bending of the wire and the following tension of the bent wire can result in displacement of the bone fragment fixed by this wire. The orientation of additional wires is assisted by observing the direction of previously inserted thin wires and half-pins and their relationship to them. This can reduce radiation exposure for the patient and surgeon by minimizing the frequency of fluoroscopic control. Therefore, do not hasten to remove the undesirably oriented wires – they can serve as useful reference points.

A towel bolster is placed between the posterior surface of the calf and the rings to eliminate sagging of the bone ends in the fracture zone, thus preserving alignment. Distraction in the frame is then performed (minimal over-distraction is desirable). Under radiological control, elimination of the mal-angulations or side displacement of the bone fragments can be performed, using one olive wire above the fracture site and another one below in the corresponding intermediate rings of the frame. The opposite end of the olive wire must also be tensioned and fixed to the corresponding ring after performing translation of the bone fragment. The end of the wire closest to the olive should be marked by a rubber plug to prevent wrongly directed withdrawal pulling during the final fixator removal procedure. We also recommend marking both ends of the olive wire differently, because a single plug may fall off during the prolonged period of external fixation.

Localization of the wire-fixator on the ring in front or behind the wire ends allows, by its tensioning, essential translation of the bone fragment to the front or back. In some cases, when it is not possible to insert the thin wire or Schanz screw through the displaced fragment, tension on the para-osseally inserted and arch-bent thin wire can move and press the fragment to the main bone fragments or to the fracture site. Not traction but pushing olive wires can also be used in this case. After such a primary positioning of this single fragment, it can be transfixed to the nearby main distal or proximal fragment. After achieving acceptable reduction, the main bone fragments must be finally fixed with additional thin wires or half-pins (one pair for each level of fixation). Inserting wires to the bone should be performed with constant awareness of the site of the neurovascular bundles. Remember: for more equal distribution of functional load-bearing, the tension on the various wires must be similar. With different levels of distraction of the wires, the more tensioned wire takes a greater load, which can result in its breakage during treatment (Fig. 3.2.1.3).

Over-distraction, required at the stage of fracture distraction, must be corrected at the end of the operative procedure. In contrast, achieving some compression of the fracture site is recommended for the treatment of patients with non-comminuted fractures and good contact between transverse-shaped main bone fragments. Warning! Over-compression of oblique-shaped bone ends and over-compression by insufficient stabilization of the bone fragments in the fixation frame or by some angular deformation of the main bone fragments can result in unwanted deformation.

Just as in unilateral frames, if the location of the proximal and distal levels of fixation (rings) is distanced from the site of the fracture as much as possible, and the intermediate rings are close to the fracture site (long lever arm fixation of distal and proximal bone fragments), rigidity of stabilization in the circular frame will be

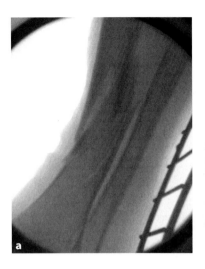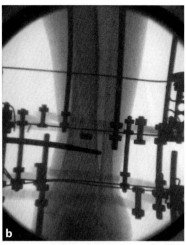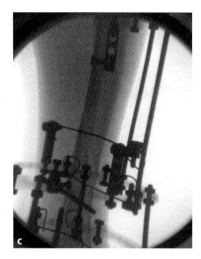

Fig. 3.2.1.3a–c. Closed reduction of the comminuted tibial fracture using distraction and fixation in the Ilizarov circular frame. **a** Radiograph on admission demonstrates comminuted displaced tibial fracture. **b,c** Closed reduction in the Ilizarov circular frame performed using olive wires

enhanced. A short frame is more comfortable for the patient but, due to a lesser level of stability of fixation, this can cause significant problems during treatment (Fig. 3.2.1.4).

A circular frame for the stabilization of femoral fractures usually includes two distal rings and one full ring placed more proximally, with an additional most proximally placed half-ring (for treating fractures in the middle or proximal third of the femoral bone, two proximal half-rings are used – a full-ring would create great discomfort at the level of the upper one-third of the thigh). Start the procedure by inserting the thin wire in the supracondylar zone of the femoral bone. This wire is introduced from the medial side in a lateral direction parallel to the articular line and to the surface of the operating table. The wire is fixed in the distal ring of the Ilizarov frame. The most proximal half-pin is introduced into the bone at the level of the lesser femoral trochanter. The assistant, holding the shin, performs manual axial distraction in the rotational alignment position and then the proximal half-pin is fixed to the proximal half-ring of the frame. The towel bolster is placed between the posterior surface of the thigh and the rings to eliminate sagging of the bone ends in the fracture zone. Then fracture distraction in the frame is performed. Additional reponating wires with olives (traction effort) and half-pins (joystick maneuver) are introduced into the bone fragments: after achieving fracture reduction, they are fixed to intermediate ("unmarried") rings of the frame. The pin configuration described by Catagni-Cattaneo ("Delta pattern"), and including one frontally oriented thin wire and two postero-medial and postero-lateral

half-pins with 60° crossing on the distal femoral ring, provides a high level of skeletal stability with minimal soft-tissue trans-fixation. Do not forget to check the rigidity of the frame itself before performing the reduction procedure!

The classic Ilizarov frame used only thin wires, but the half-pins became more widely used bone-fixation elements in later generations of circular fixation frames, especially in femoral fixation frames. At the present time, most circular frames use half-pin fixation in the proximal part of the femoral bone and thin wires (or a combination of wires and half-pins) in the distal part of the femoral bone. Trans-fixation of significant muscle bulk is unavoidable when applying external femoral fixation and frequently causes restriction of movement of the knee joint, not only during the external fixation period, but also after removing the fixation frames. Lengthy intensive physiotherapeutic treatment is needed to restore knee movement, and sometimes closed manipulation under anesthesia followed by continuous passive motions machine treatment or arthroscopy to lyze intra-articular knee adhesions may be required. More extensive surgical treatment, such as quadricepsplasty (stepwise release of the knee and quadriceps muscle – the Judet quadricepsplasty in the Paley modification [104]), may be required. To prevent this severe complication, we use the following tactics:

1. Avoid inserting the thin wires and half-pins through muscle-tendon units.
2. When inserting wires near the joint line which cross from the extensor to the flexor surface, flexion of the knee is necessary until the wire crosses the bone; the knee must be extended during the passage of the

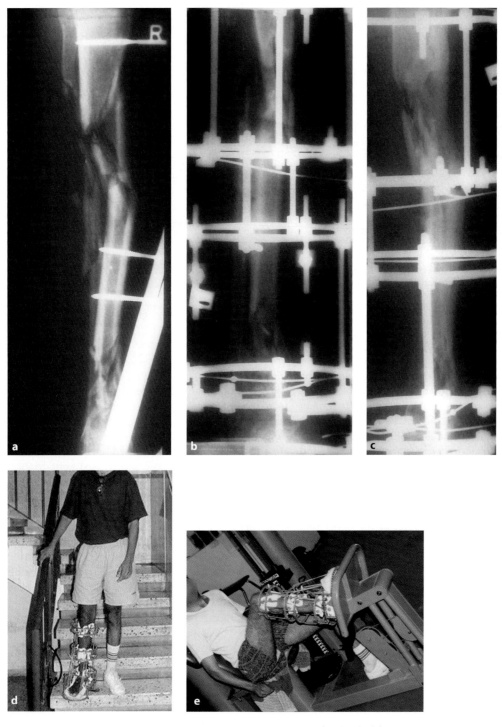

Fig. 3.2.1.4a–i. A 24-year-old who sustained an open multicomminuted right tibial fracture with extensive damage to soft tissues caused by the blast of a land mine. On admission, there was associated full motor and sensory deficit to right leg and foot. **a** Emergency treatment included radical debridement of the wounds, fasciotomy and unilateral external stabilization using AO tubular frame. **b,c** Three weeks later, unilateral tubular fixator was converted to Ilizarov circular frame, and closed reduction of the fracture was performed. The radiographic appearance after reduction demonstrates acceptable axis of the tibial bone. **d,e** Early functional treatment, including functional weight-bearing, was started immediately after conversion to a circular fixation frame. Spontaneous recovery of the peripheral nerve injuries was observed 7 months later. Clinical appearance of functional weight-bearing on the injured lower limb. **f–i** *see next page*

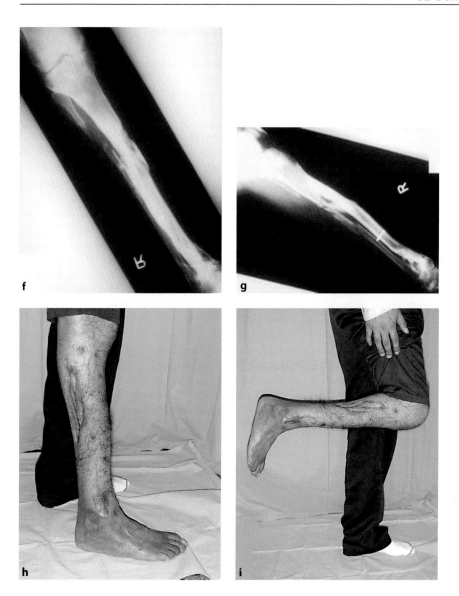

Fig. 3.2.1.4a–i. *(continued)* **f,g** Ilizarov fixator was removed after 12 months of fixation. The final radiological appearance on long-term follow-up after 24 months demonstrates solid bone healing of the tibial fracture with the presence of a broken fragment of the half-pin incorporated into the bone. **h,i** Clinical view at follow-up after 24 months. Good clinical result; patient returned to his job as a professional military officer

wire through the flexors. This produces a definite reserve of soft tissues near the joint and diminishes mechanical obstacles to joint motion during external fixation.

3. Proper patient education, early active and passive motions of the joints of the operated limb, and early functional loading, including weight-bearing, must be a rule.

4. Effective analgesia in the postoperative period allows early and greater functional treatment.

5. Avoid prolonged fixed positioning of the limbs, especially full extension or flexion. It is essential to preserve some flexion (10°–15°) in the knee joint at all times, including during postoperative limb elevation.

In order to perform this transition efficiently with minimal additional trauma, we use the inserted half-pins from the primary tubular external fixator that were applied in the emergency treatment phase. It is desirable to preserve half-pins without signs of local infection, half-pins with good fixation to the bone, half-pins in the "correct localization", i.e., the half-pins which do not transfix the muscles and tendons and the joint capsule. Tension of the soft tissues around half-pins, restricting motions in the adjoining joints, requires their re-insertion. We add more tension wires and additional half-pins to correct inadequate positioning of bone fragments and to provide final stabile fixation. The number of rings, transosseous wires and half-pins can vary, according to fracture patterns and complexity. Attention must be paid to releasing the bridged joints as soon as possible, in order to preserve their range of movement. A fracture reduction technique without open exposure is possible in most patients; the circular device can greatly facilitate reduction and successful ligamentotaxis aided by thin wires with olives as pullers or pushers, changing distances and angulation, and

inter-orientation of the rings in the external fixation frame [121, 125, 126]. Moreover, the use of half-pins as "joysticks" to transfer and reduce relatively large bone fragments can also be useful in closed reduction procedures. Before insertion of reponating thin wires or half-pins, the soft tissue mass and the skin must be so positioned as to prevent ensuing tension of soft tissues around the fixation elements.

In patients in whom attempted closed reduction was unsuccessful, especially for treating intra-articular fractures in which precise anatomical reduction is needed, open reduction must be performed, while keeping in mind the balance between the potential positive effects of articular reconstruction in very severe injuries and the potential complications in restoring articular anatomy. A careful, atraumatic technique that minimizes direct injury to the soft tissues during definitive fracture surgery is crucial [136]. Open reduction of bone fragments in the presence of an external fixation frame allows a lesser surgical approach and, accordingly, is accompanied by less soft-tissue traumatization while facilitating distraction, ligamentotaxis, and axial alignment with thin wires with olives, including their application for closed reduction in the external fixation frame to achieve final reduction (Fig. 3.2.1.5).

Reduction is usually significantly simplified in the treatment of open fractures with exposed bone ends. Open reduction is achieved through the wound and maintained with clamps or by applying thin wires through the reduced bone fragments. Then the pre-assembled frame is applied on the injured limb segment and thin wires and half-pins are introduced into the bone fragments according to the fracture configuration and soft-tissue condition. The clamps and wires of the temporary fixation can be removed once stable fixation of the fragments in the circular/hybrid external fixation frame has been achieved.

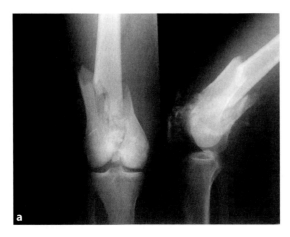

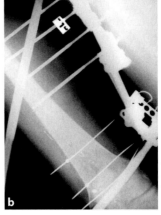

Fig. 3.2.1.5a,b. A 21-year-old soldier who sustained a distal femoral fracture caused by a grenade blast. **a** Radiograph on admission demonstrates comminuted intra-articular displaced femoral fracture. **b** Post-operative radiograph demonstrates anatomical reduction of the fracture with external fixation using a hybrid frame with half-pins and olive wires

For stabilization of bone fragments after open reduction of the fracture, we use thin wires and olive wires, tensioned and fixed to the external frame. Additional separate thin wires can also be used to fix several simple small bone fragments. To prevent migration of these wires, it is desirable to fix them to the corresponding rings of the frame. In treating patients with good soft-tissue coverage over the fracture site, it is possible to produce fixation of the single peri-articular bone fragment using additional cannulated screws. To prevent complications, such as the spread of superficial pin tract infection and its extension into the deep tissues and bone, contact between the screws and thin wires of the external fixation frame must be avoided (Fig. 3.2.1.6, Fig. 3.2.1.7).

Insertion of the thin wires not only in the plane of the ring but also in various other planes increases the level of stability of fixation in the external frame. Introduction of wires into the bone from various sites on the ring can also create additional stability. The bone becomes significantly weakened by insertion of wires from different sites but in one plane of the ring. That can cause a pathological fracture at this site. Increased stability of fracture fixation can also be achieved by a wider use of olive wires. All these procedures are usually performed under fluoroscopic imaging control of the placement of the half-pins and thin wires, skeletal alignment and fracture reduction. The final check is by two standard antero-posterior and lateral radiographs (Fig. 3.2.1.8).

When good bone fragment reduction is achieved by primary skeletal stabilization, it is desirable to preserve the alignment during the conversion from the tubular external fixation frame to the circular Ilizarov device [77]. We recommend performing the following sequence of actions for this purpose. The more distant tube of the double tubular frame must be moved in the direction of the outer ends of the half-pins and strongly fixed. The tube placed nearer the injured limb segment can then be removed. Thus, an adequate place for mounting a circular external fixation frame around the fixed segment is provided, preserving the previously achieved bone fragment position. The half-pins of the primary tubular external fixator are attached to the circular frame by fixing them to the corresponding rings. To include the half-pin in the circular Ilizarov frame without losing, even temporarily, its importance for the fixation properties of the primary tubular frame, we use the following simple technical method. To the proximal ring toward the half-pin, we attach the supporting masculine end or post-feminine end. The half-pin is fastened to the supporting masculine end or post-feminine end using an encircling buckle. Some additional thin wires and half-pins are introduced to the bone fragments and only now, after ensuring the stability of the main bone fragments, is the primary tubular external fixation frame removed. The hazard of secondary displacement of the bone fragments with loss of alignment and additional traumatization to the soft tissues is thus avoided; the timing of the operative procedure can be shortened, and exposure to irradiation of the patient and operating staff is also diminished. Moreover, part of this procedure (mounting of the circular external frame on the base of the available half-pins of the AO tubular external fixator) does not need anesthesia and can be performed directly in the hospital ward, saving operating room time (significant in mass casualty situations) (Fig. 3.2.1.9).

For the functional restoration of the ankle joint in peri-articular fractures in the distal third of the legs, anatomical reconstruction of both tibial and fibular bones is needed. The importance of the anatomical reduction and rigid internal fixation of the fractured lower third of the fibular bone is emphasized in some publications. It is often recommended to begin the reconstruction procedure with open reduction and stable internal fixation of the fibular bone as a good anatomical reference point for restoration of the length and final reconstruction of the distal tibial bone. The method of fibular plating and sometimes additional lag-screw techniques are recommended in most cases for this reason. However, after high-energy trauma, soft-tissue conditions often exclude the possibility of internal fracture fixation which needs an additional incision and coverage of the implanted internal fixation device, as well as the fracture site.

The method of thin wire fixation in the circular/hybrid external fixation frames allows stabilization of severe comminuted complex fractures in the distal third of the tibial bone (including pylon fractures) and is well established in the treatment of these challenging injuries. The presence of the fixation plate on the fibular bone surface can considerably confuse the insertion of the distal thin wire across both tibial and fibular bones that are essential for increasing fixation stability, especially in treating low meta-epiphyseal fractures of the tibial bone with comminution of its lateral cortex.

In tibial fractures treated by external fixation techniques, the necessity of rigid fibular fixation has been questioned. This can result in delayed or non-union of the tibial bone, with varus deformity of the fracture site. Rigid fixation of the fibular bone, provided by plating and screw fixation, is an obstacle in the use of the Ilizarov method; it diminishes its unique ability in exerting ongoing dynamic influence on the tibial bone fracture site [123]. Rigid fixation of the fibula deprives the Ilizarov method of its multiple possibilities, converting it into a simple external fixation device (Fig. 3.2.1.10).

Moreover, the possibility of large bone defect filling and lower limb length restoration using a method of callotasis is excluded by the presence of rigid fibular fixation. Concerning this Williams (1998) wrote: "Open

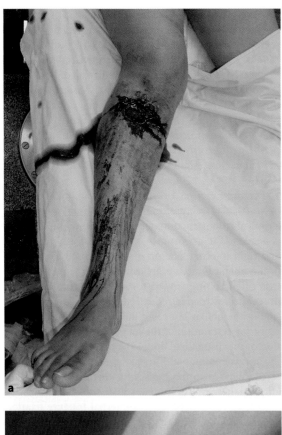

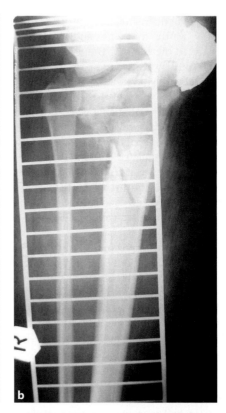

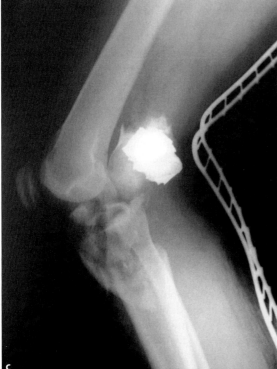

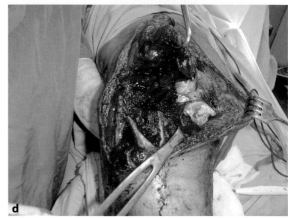

Fig. 3.2.1.6a–p. A 28-year-old female. This victim of a road traffic accident sustained an open fracture of the right tibia with a large foreign body in the knee joint. **a–c** The appearance of the injury, both clinical (severe valgus knee deformity with laceration over proximal third of the leg) and radiographic (severe comminuting of proximal third of the tibia with large foreign body in the knee joint). **d** Surgical exploration of the wound. Clinical photo demonstrates severe intra-articular comminution of the proximal third of the tibial bone. **e–p** *see next pages*

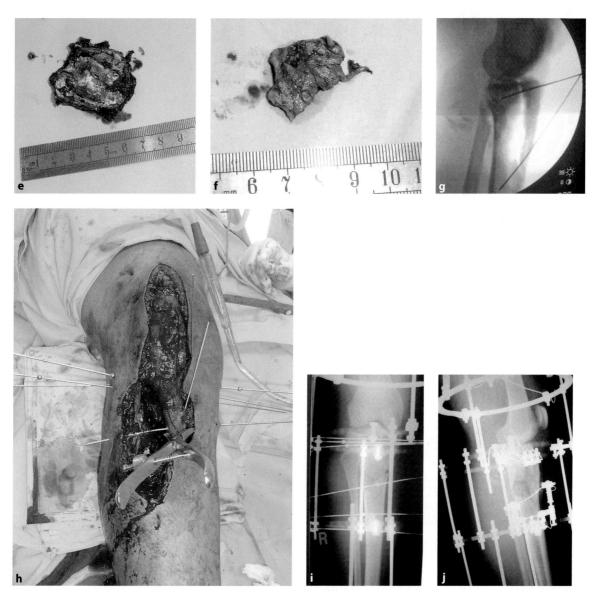

Fig. 3.2.1.6a–p. *(continued)* **e** Metal foreign body is removed from the knee joint. **f** Large de-attached fragment of the skin found in the knee joint and removed. **g,h** Open reduction and provisory thin wire fixation of the bone fragments is performed. Intra-operative radiological and clinical views. **i–j** Three weeks later. Radiological and clinical views. Ilizarov eternal fixation of the tibial fracture with temporary knee bridging. Skin grafting was performed on the granulated surface of the wound. **k–p** *see next page*

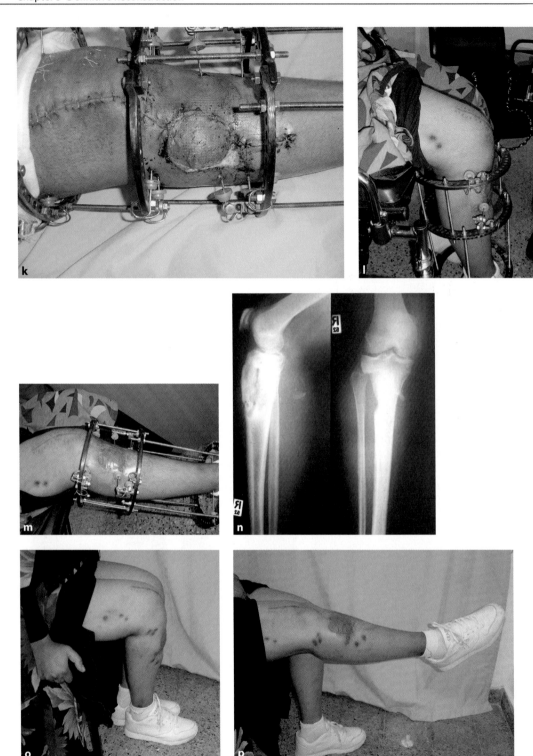

Fig. 3.2.1.6a–p. *(continued)* **k** Three weeks later. Radiological and clinical views. Ilizarov eternal fixation of the tibial fracture with temporary knee bridging. Skin grafting was performed on the granulated surface of the wound. **l,m** Clinical view 1 month after injury. Knee mobilization after removing the femoral ring of the Ilizarov device and freeing the joint. The Ilizarov external fixator is definitively removed 6 months after injury. **n–p** Radiological and clinical control 1 year after injury. Radiographically, good bone healing with restored tibial articular surface

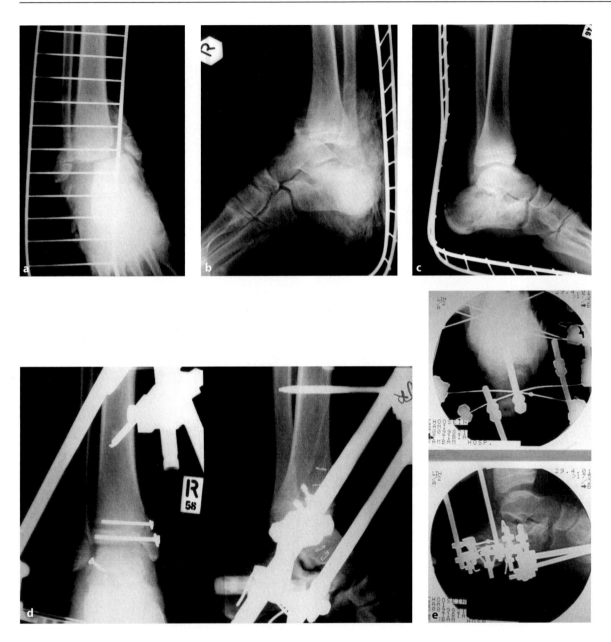

Fig. 3.2.1.7a–o. A 15-year-old male with bilateral lower limb injuries due to a fall from the third floor. **a–c** Radiographs on admission. Bimalleolar displaced right ankle fracture and talar bone fracture; comminuted left calcaneal fracture. **d,e** Minimal internal fixation of medial malleolus and talar bone using screws; additional hybrid external tibio-calcaneal bridging is performed on the right lower limb. Ilizarov external fixation of the left calcaneal fracture is performed. Control post-operative radiographs of both lower limbs. **f–o** *see next pages*

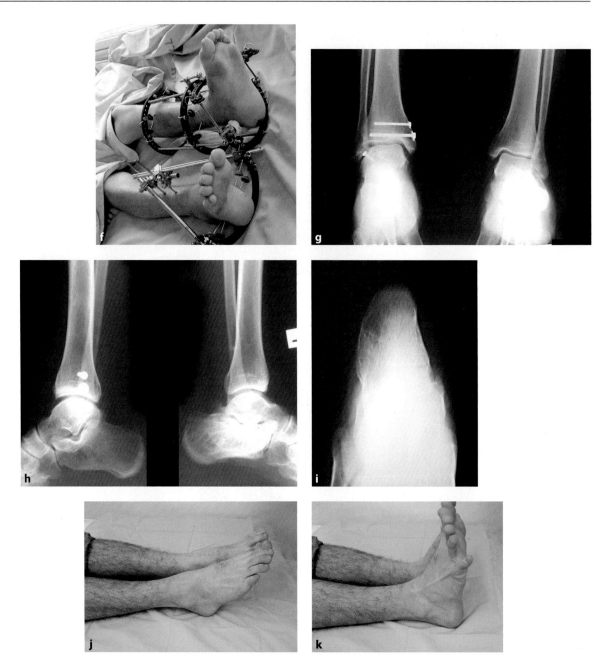

Fig. 3.2.1.7a–o. *(continued)* **f** Post-operative clinical appearance of the lower limbs. **g–i** Radiological examination on follow-up 2 years after injury. Note radiological appearance of solid bone consolidation in good alignment. **j–k** Clinical appearance on follow-up 2 years after injury. Good post-operative range of ankle and subtalar motions of both operated legs. **l–o** *see next page*

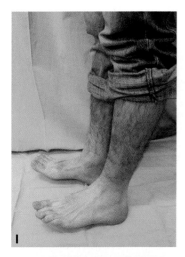

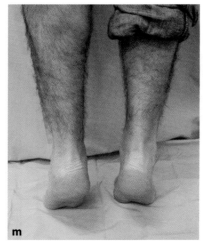

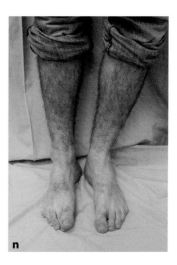

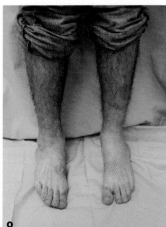

Fig. 3.2.1.7a–o. *(continued)* **l–o** Clinical appearance on follow-up 2 years after injury. Good post-operative range of ankle and subtalar motions of both operated legs

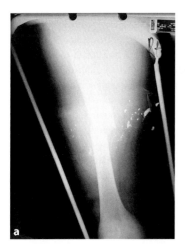

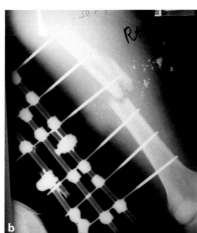

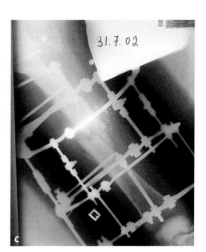

Fig. 3.2.1.8a–j. A 27-year-old male with open fracture right femur Gustilo–Anderson type IIIA due to high-velocity gun-shot injury. **a** X-rays on admission demonstrate a comminuted femoral shaft fracture. Note the foreign bodies in the fracture zone. **b** On admission the patient had primary debridement of wounds. Skeletal stabilization was performed using unilateral tubular AO external fixation frame. Control post-operative radiograph of the leg fixed by unilateral frame. **c** Radiological picture after conversion of unilateral tubular to circular Ilizarov frame. Note good axial alignment with minimal lateral translation of bone fragments. **d–e** *see next page*

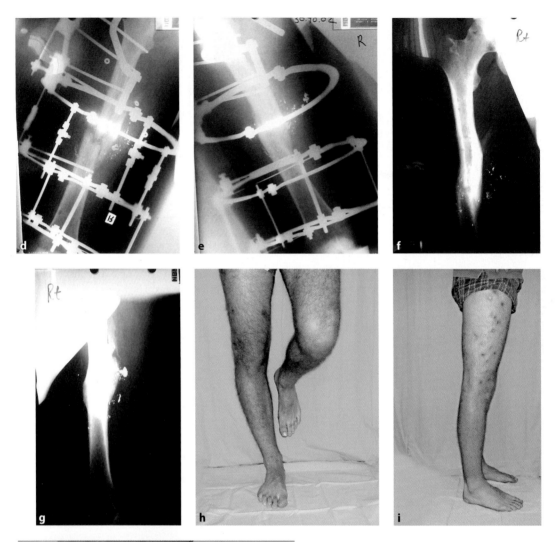

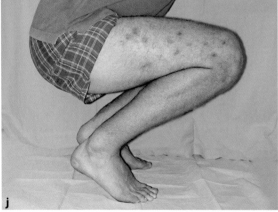

Fig. 3.2.1.8a–j. *(continued)* **d** Radiological picture after conversion of unilateral tubular to circular Ilizarov frame. Note good axial alignment with minimal lateral translation of bone fragments. **e** Early full weight-bearing allowed during the stabilization period in the Ilizarov external fixation frame. Note that threaded rods above the fracture zone have been removed for clinical testing of the solidity of the union and better radiological image in the final stage of external fixation. Radiological signs of solid bone healing. **f,g** Radiological examination on follow-up 2 years after removing the Ilizarov external fixation frame. Note radiological appearance of solid bone consolidation in good alignment. **h–j** Clinical appearance on follow-up 2 years after removing the Ilizarov fixation frame. Full range of movement of the knee joint

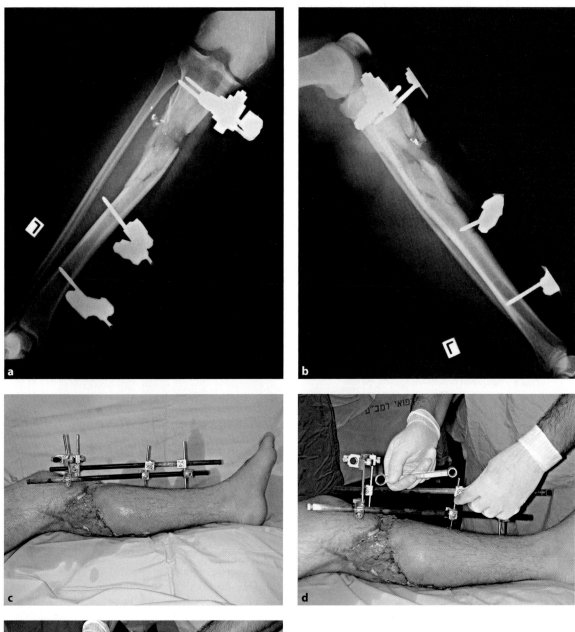

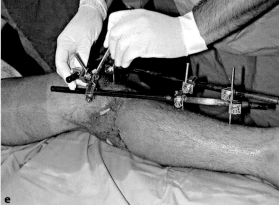

Fig. 3.2.1.9a–t. A 27-year-old male with open fracture of right proximal tibia with soft-tissue and bone loss due to combat gunshot injury. Surgical exploration of the wound, debridement and external fixation using a unilateral tubular frame were performed on admission. Five days later, wound coverage was performed with local rotational soft-tissue flap and skin graft. **a,b** Radiological appearance after re-alignment and stabilization using unilateral external fixation frame. Note proximal tibial bone loss. **c** Clinical appearance of the lower limb after soft-tissue wound healing. **d–e** Clinical photos demonstrate steps of "lateralization" in unilateral external fixation frame. **f–t** *see next page*

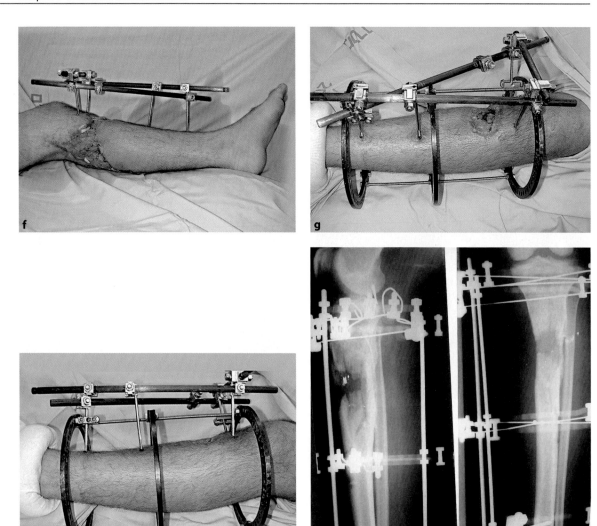

Fig. 3.2.1.9a–t. *(continued)* **f** Clinical photos demonstrate steps of "lateralization" in unilateral external fixation frame. **g,h** Assembly of circular external fixation frame using half-pins of the primary tubular fixation frame. During this procedure, fracture fragments are fixed by the primary unilateral frame. **i** Radiological appearance of fracture fixation using circular Ilizarov frame. **j–o** *see next pages*

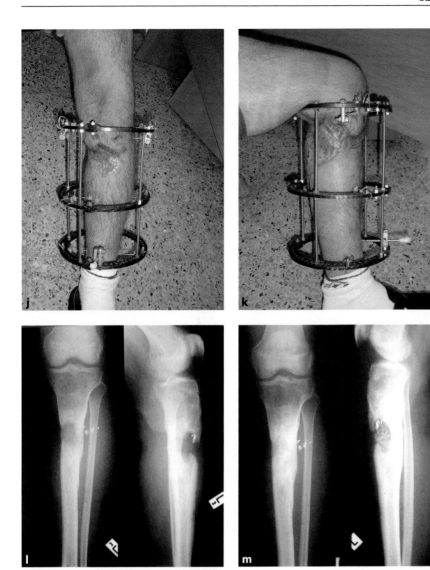

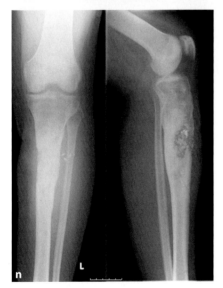

Fig. 3.2.1.9a–t. *(continued)* **j,k** Clinical photos of functional treatment and weight-bearing in Ilizarov fixation frame. **l** Ilizarov fixation frame removed after 6 months of external fixation. Radiograph demonstrates partial bone healing with bone defect on anterior part of proximal tibia. **m** Debridement and removing fibrous tissue from bone defect with filling of the defect with calcium-phosphate chips. **n** Radiograph 6 months later demonstrates integration process of calcium-phosphate cement. **o–t** *see next page*

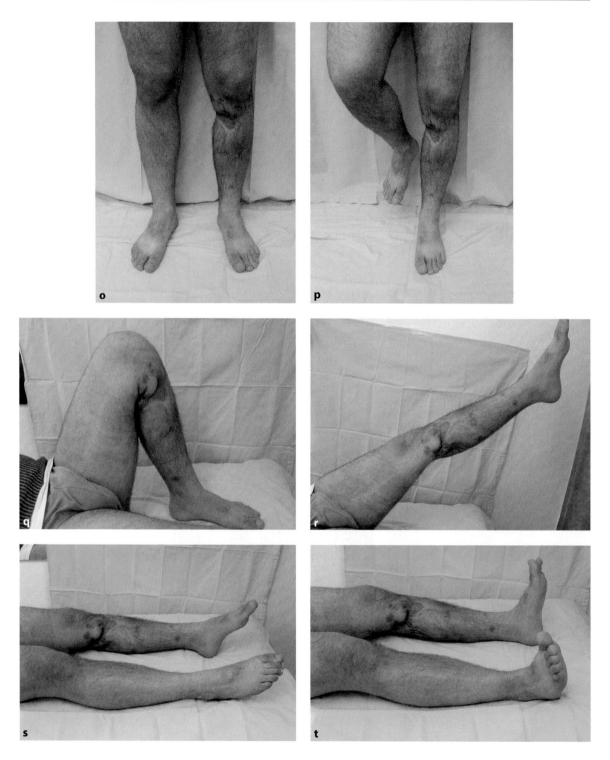

Fig. 3.2.1.9a–t. *(continued)* **o–t** Functional results at follow-up 2 years after trauma

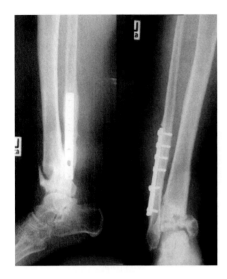

Fig. 3.2.1.10. A 36-year-old male with open fracture of distal tibial and fibular bones Gustilo–Anderson type IIIA due to a fall from 5 m. Open reduction and internal fixation of the fibula by plating was performed. The tibia was fixed using an Ilizarov external fixation frame. The possibility of an active influence of the Ilizarov frame on the comminuted tibial fracture with bone defect was diminished by the rigid internal fixation of the fibula and following solid union of the fibula. Radiological appearance of distal tibial non-union with varus deformity, united fibular fracture after internal fixation by plating

reduction and internal fixation of the fibula in tibial pla-fond fractures treated with external fixation that spans the ankle is associated with a significant rate of complications, and good clinical results may be obtained without fixing the fibula" [143]. Thus, in treating these patients, we perform a closed fibular bone reposition in the Ilizarov circular frame, utilizing the method of ligamentotaxis with olive wires for reduction and fixation. When treating patients in whom open fibular reposition is needed, bone stabilization in the achieved position of reduction of the fibular bone can be performed with intramedullary placed (antegrade or retrograde) thin rods or wires.

The absence of rigid fixation on the lateral (fibular) column preserves the possibility of an active influence on the medial (tibial) column and of performing compression/distraction forces using Ilizarov external circular frames during the period of external fixation. For treating patients with such distal tibial fractures, including pylon fractures, we use a pre-constructed circular fixation frame consisting of a proximal block of two rings for tibial shaft fixation, one more distally placed free ring above the meta-epiphyseal level, and a foot ring. Distraction is performed between the tibial block and the foot ring for ligamentotaxis and re-alignment of the bone fragments. Trans-fixation of the bone fragments

using thin wires connected to the free intermediate ring is performed after achieving a radiological picture of anatomical reduction. Additional olive wires can be an effective tool for performing closed reduction of residual displaced bone fragments. If the attempt at closed reduction is unsuccessful, the fracture must be reduced surgically with stabilization of the fragments using olive wires and/or cannulated screws (Fig. 3.2.1.11).

Sometimes, even after successful closed reconstruction of the intra-articular surface of the tibial bone, metaphyseal fragments of the anterior tibial crest remain unreduced and depressed. This condition may cause delayed fracture union, demanding an additional bone grafting procedure. A closed reduction technique for the elevation of a depressed cortical fragment using a percutaneously inserted half-pin as a joystick can be a simple solution to this problem, avoiding additional open surgery (Fig. 3.2.1.12).

High-energy injuries are associated with a marked tendency to severe post-traumatic swelling of the injured limb. This, and the necessity to preserve a sufficient space for the treatment of soft-tissue wounds, dictates the need to apply larger diameter rings than is usually recommended in assembling the circular frame in standard situations (recommended distance between skin of fixed limb segment and frame is about 2 cm). Moreover, increasing the ring diameter results in reduction of the bone fragment fixation stability. The longer the wire lever length and the larger the ring diameter, the less the stability of the fracture fragment fixation. To eliminate this undesirable effect, we recommend, when using large diameter frames, the insertion of one or two more thin wires or half-pins into each of the main bone fragments (Fig. 3.2.1.13, Fig. 3.2.1.14).

The number of rings in the external frame is directly proportional to the degree of system stability and, correspondingly, to the reliability of fracture fixation. The standard Ilizarov fixation frame usually contains four rings, two per fixed bone segment. One or even two additional rings are needed for stable fixation and active influence on isolated large bone fragments when treating patients suffering from segmental fractures. The number of connection threaded rods between rings is also directly proportional to the frame stability; at least four rods must be used on each level. In the assembly of a frame including large diameter rings, one or two more threaded connection rods must be placed between the rings. The rods should be oriented perpendicularly to the rings; oblique or bent positioning of the connecting rods must be eliminated. The frame stability is inversely proportional to the distance between the rings and, consequently, additional threaded rods must be placed at a relatively large distance between the rings.

In the standard configuration of the Ilizarov frame, two wires per ring are usually used. The greatest stability is obtained with a 90° crossing of the ring wires. Practically, to avoid unnecessary soft-tissue trans-fixation, the

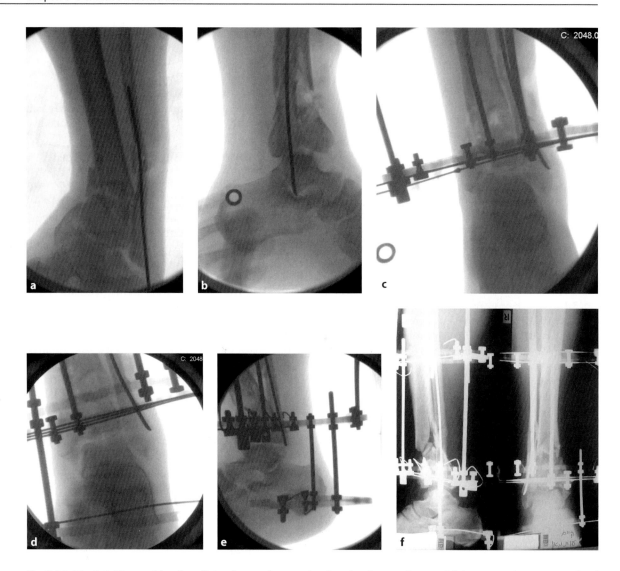

Fig. 3.2.1.11a–l. A 29-year-old male suffering from comminuted right pylon fracture due to a fall from 6 m. This patient suffered from Behçet's syndrome with skin involvement including the right lower limb. Immediate closed reduction of the fractures with Ilizarov external fixation was performed. **a,b** The operative procedure was started with closed reduction and intramedullary fixation of the fibular bone using a thin nail. Radiograph after performing fibular internal fixation. **c** Intra-operative radiological picture after performing closed reduction and Ilizarov external fixation of the tibial bone. **d,e** Additional trans-ankle fixation is performed to increase fixation stability due to short and comminuted distal tibial fragments. **f** Radiological examination 10 weeks after injury demonstrates signs of very weak consolidation process with good alignment of bone fragments. **g–l** *see next page*

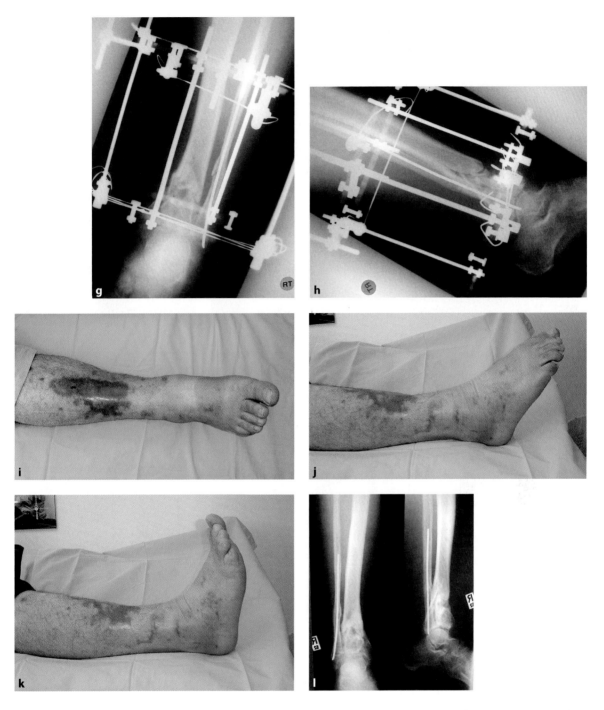

Fig. 3.2.1.11a–l. *(continued)* **g,h** Radiological examination 16 weeks after injury demonstrates signs of partial consolidation of the tibial bone. **i–k** After 6 months of external fixation, the Ilizarov frame was removed. Clinical photos at 3 months after removing the external fixation frame demonstrate good range of active motions in the ankle joint. **l** Radiological appearance at 3 months after removing the external fixation frame demonstrates bone healing of the tibial and fibular fracture in good alignment with preservation of the articular surface

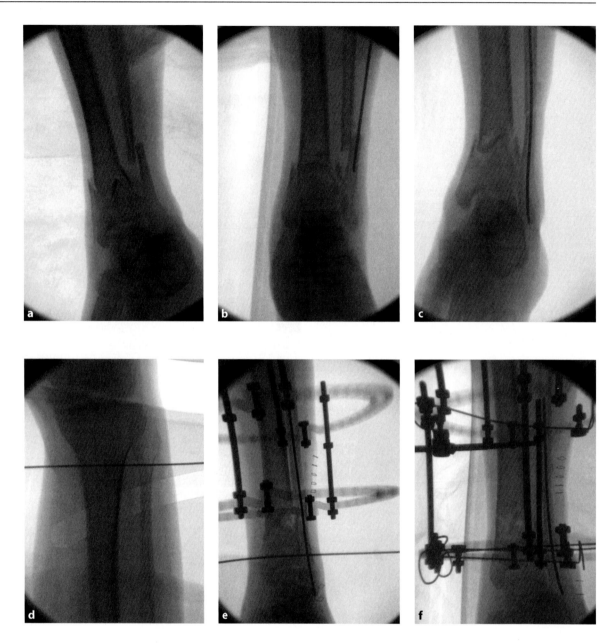

Fig. 3.2.1.12a–i. A 36-year-old male suffering from comminuted left distal tibial and fibular fractures due to a fall from 7 m. Immediate closed reduction of the fractures with Ilizarov external fixation was performed. **a** Radiograph on admission demonstrates severe bone comminuting and displacement. **b** The operative procedure is started with open reduction and intramedullary fixation of the fibular bone using a thin nail. Radiograph demonstrates the retrograde technique of intramedullary fibular fixation. **c** Intraoperative radiological photo after performing reduction and intramedullary fixation of the fibular bone. **d** Proximal thin wire is introduced to the tibial bone. Note its placement parallel to the knee joint articular line. **e** Radiological picture after insertion of the distal thin wire to the tibial bone. Note the radiological signs of the pre-assembled Ilizarov fixation frame. **f** Closed reduction and fixation of the tibial fracture in the external fixation frame. Note severe comminuting of the distal tibial bone with depressed anterior cortical fragment on the control X-ray examination. **g–i** *see next page*

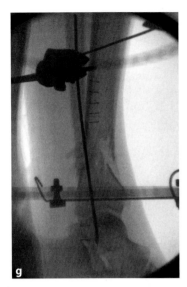
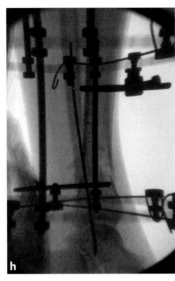
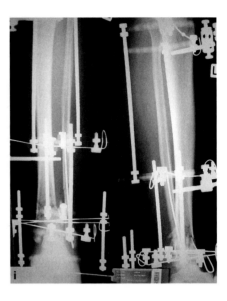

Fig. 3.2.1.12a–i. *(continued)* **g** Closed reduction and fixation of the tibial fracture in the external fixation frame. Note severe comminuting of the distal tibial bone with depressed anterior cortical fragment on the control X-ray examination. **h** Elevation of the anterior cortical fragment is performed using an additional half-pin as joystick. Intra-operative radiological picture demonstrates reduction of the cortical fragment. **i** Control radiography 1 month later demonstrates acceptable position of the bone fragments

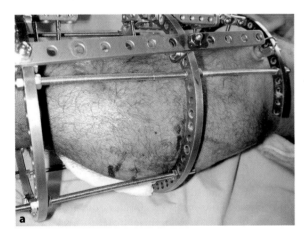
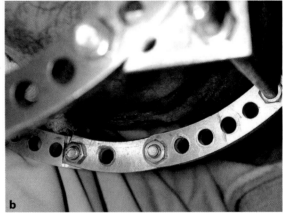
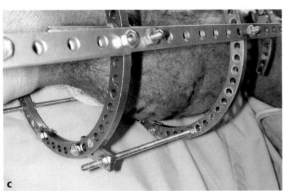

Fig. 3.2.1.13a–c. a Clinical appearance of local skin pressure due to severe post-traumatic swelling of the injured limb. **b** The fixator's pressure on the skin is released by adding a short connection plate, inserted between half-rings, in order to enlarge the inner diameter of the ring. Note local signs of constrained skin. **c** Clinical appearance of the injured limb after solving the problem

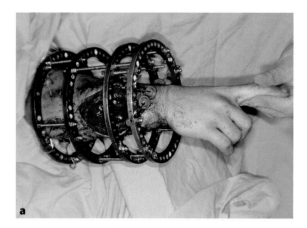
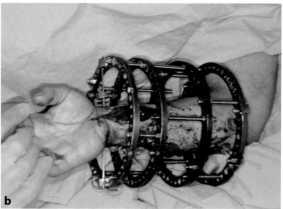

Fig. 3.2.1.14a,b. Clinical appearance of large external fixation frame used for stabilization of forearm fractures in a patient with severe blast injury

wire crossing angle is different, considerably less than recommended. Thus, the stability is decreased, especially when angulation between the wires is less than 45°. Using thin wires with olives can raise the level of mechanical bone stability in the fixation frame. A similar effect can be achieved by using large diameter half-pins; for fixation of femoral or tibial bones, we usually use 6-mm diameter half-pins. When using large diameter rings, it is very important to remember the need for two-level fixation of each main bone fragment. Internal stability provided by direct contact of main bone fragments can contribute to the general stability provided by the external fixator. In transverse fractures, shearing forces can be controlled by applying simple compression across the fracture. But victims of high-energy injuries, especially war injuries, suffer from comminuted fractures, often with some bone loss. In such situations, stability must be provided by the fixation frame itself in the early stages of treatment. Consequently, some additional fixation elements (thin wires, half-pins) must be added to increase the level of stabilization of each main bone fragment and, correspondingly, the whole fixation frame itself.

It is possible to avoid excessive and uncomfortable fixation frame enlargement by the asymmetrical placement of the fixed limb segment into the circular fixation frame, preserving a greater distance between the skin and the inner part of the ring only on the inferior surface of the limb, taking into account the likelihood of swelling and spreading of the posterior aspect of the thigh, calf, arm, and forearm. However, even when using asymmetric positioning of the injured limb segment in the external fixation frame, it is necessary to ensure symmetrical fixation of the distal bone fragment with regard to the proximal one. Remember that asymmetrical positioning of the limb segment, especially asym-

metrical localization of the bone to the center of the frame, can diminish the level of stability of fixation.

One of the primary advantages of external fixation in the circular Ilizarov frame is the ongoing ability to actively influence the position of the bone fragments during the entire period of external fixation. This allows the closed, gradual, atraumatic, and pain-free final alignment of the bone fragments, avoiding the necessity of attaining an immediate final reduction surgically, necessitating potentially traumatizing, one-moment soft-tissue tension around the bone and causing possible vascular disturbance of the bone fragments, especially undesirable in high-energy injuries (Fig. 3.2.1.15).

Returning to the axiom that the condition of the soft tissues is the determining factor in treating patients suffering from high-energy trauma, we emphasize that fixation of the injured limb in the circular frame establishes optimal conditions for the soft tissues in the early definitive phases of the treatment process. Circular frames enable continuous elevation of the injured segment and afford all-round mechanical protection, shielding the limb evenly on all sides from pressure and avoiding gravitational impingement on the skin and soft tissues on the inferior surface of the limb. Moreover, it may be unnecessary to apply circular pressure bandages when using this method. Local pressure on the wound, if needed, can be achieved by placing a pressure cotton pad between the wound and the ring of the frame, eliminating undesirable pressure on other areas near the injured segment. This can be a useful method of treating complex injuries, such as burns, especially circular burns, compartment syndrome, and post-fasciotomy conditions.

Additional inspection of the assembled fixation frame must be performed in the final stage of the opera-

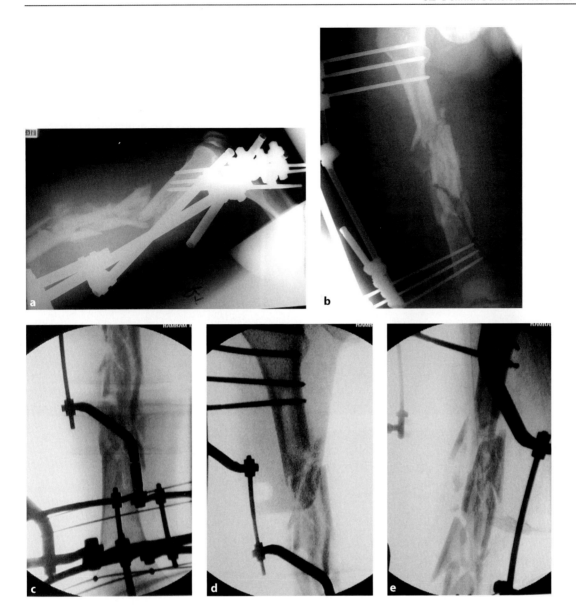

Fig. 3.2.1.15a–l. A 32-year-old male with open fracture of the right femur, Gustilo–Anderson type IIIA, and penetrating head injury due to a high-velocity gun-shot. Immediate debridement and external fixation using a unilateral tubular frame was performed on admission. **a** Control post-operative radiographs after primary skeletal stabilization in the unilateral fixation frame. Note severe comminuting of the femoral bone in the fracture zone. **b–e** Six days later, conversion of unilateral frame to Ilizarov circular fixation frame was performed. Note that proximal half-pins of the initial unilateral fixator are used in assembling the final Ilizarov frame. Radiological appearance after conversion of the unilateral tubular frame to the Ilizarov frame demonstrates good axial alignment of the multi-comminuted femoral fracture. **f–l** *see next pages*

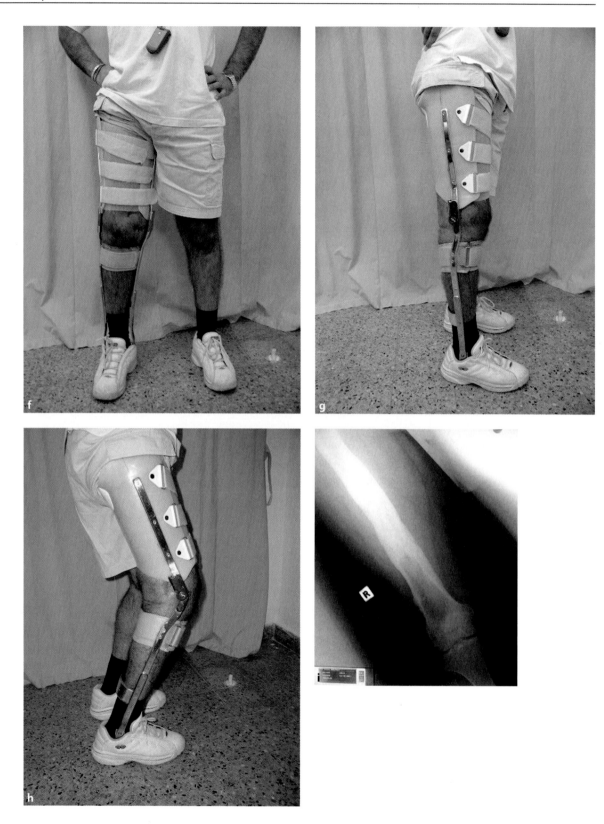

Fig. 3.2.1.15a–l. *(continued)* **f–h** Early full weight-bearing was allowed during entire period of stabilization in the Ilizarov external fixation frame. The Ilizarov frame was removed after 7 months in view of radiological signs of consolidation. Additional fixation of the lower limb using a hinged plastic brace was continued for another 4 months. Clinical appearance of the hinged plastic brace. **i** Radiological examination on follow-up 2 years after removing Ilizarov external fixation frame. Note radiological appearance of the solid bone consolidation in good alignment. **j–l** *see next page*

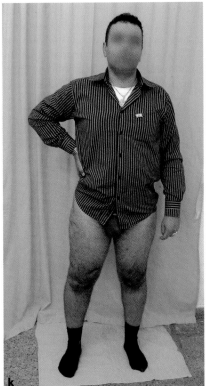

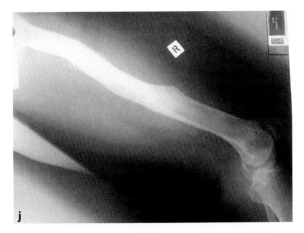

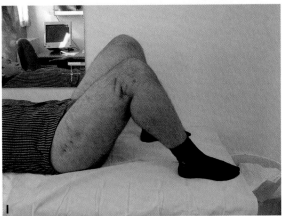

Fig. 3.2.1.15a–l. *(continued)* **j** Radiological examination on follow-up 2 years after removing Ilizarov external fixation frame. Note radiological appearance of the solid bone consolidation in good alignment. **k,l** Clinical appearance on follow-up 2 years after removing the Ilizarov fixation frame

tive procedure, checking the degree of its stability and also the stability of the fracture fixation, and checking and eliminating skin and soft-tissue tension around fixation elements. Unreleased skin tension may be the cause of severe postoperative pain and joint stiffness, and can lead to local skin necrosis and pin tract infection [81].

3.2.2 Hybrid Frames (Modular Combinations in Various Types of External Fixation Devices)

The extensive damage caused by high-energy injuries requires a flexible approach. The simultaneous use of different external fixation systems, such as tubular, circular (Ilizarov) or hybrid, is often the modular solution to this problem. Such hybrid modular fixation systems, using a relatively small number of components, provide many options for fixation frames.

It is desirable to use the merits of the unilateral tubular external fixator in choosing a method for final fracture fixation: simplicity, ease of use, less trans-fixation of soft tissues, accessibility to the soft tissues of the injured limb segment, and positioning of the limb, especially with external fixation of proximal femoral and humeral fractures. At the same time, the fixation device must possess the unique merits of the circular external fixator, ongoing correction during the entire period of external fixation, with reliability of fixation, sufficient for full weight-bearing, even in patients with multi-comminuted fractures and severe bone defects. Other merits are the possibility of active manipulation in the fracture zone, and the possibility of filling significant bone defects without using traumatic methods of bone grafting. The objective of the hybrid external fixation device is to combine the desirable properties of different kinds of external fixators. The hybrid system is minimally invasive and requires less trans-fixation of the surrounding soft tissues as compared to the standard thin wire circular fixation frame. It combines the advantages of both unilateral cantilever and ring/wire external fixation systems, and provides a good solution for metaphyseal and intra-articular fractures with severe soft-tissue damage.

The concomitant use of different kinds of fixation frames creates problems related to the assembling of the diverse parts. To solve problems generated by the simultaneous use of different external fixation combinations, "transitional blocks" for use between systems were developed, such as modified AO single adjustable clamps which allow the tubular rod of the external fixator system to be connected to the ring of the Ilizarov set [40]. However, the diversity and severity of tissue damage due to high-energy injuries creates a demand for various simple and reliable methods of intersystem fixation for the variety of external fixation frames. We have used several simple methods for joining various

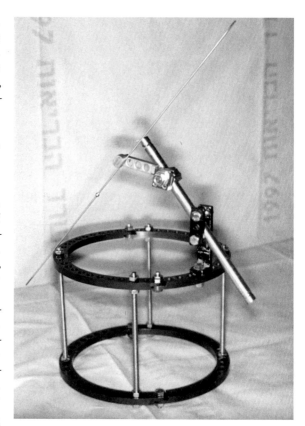

Fig. 3.2.2.1. Joining the tensioned thin wire to the Ilizarov male clamp, adjusted to the tubular rod of the external fixator. *Lerner et al. Modular use of external fixation configurations for treatment of complex and severely injured limbs. Eur J Trauma 2003; 29:108–111 [77] (© Urban & Vogel. Reproduced with permission)*

components of different external fixation systems, using only parts from standard sets, thereby both simplifying and shortening the emergency operation, and eliminating the need for additional transitional blocks. We generally use combinations of the AO/ASIF tubular fixator and the Ilizarov circular frame [77]. In the treatment of some patients, certain components of standard hybrid fixators are also included. Our mechanical procedures are as follows:

1. Joining the tensioned thin wire to the tubular rod of the unilateral external fixator. The wire is connected in the usual way to the male clamp of the Ilizarov system, which is attached to the AO single clamp. Thus it is possible to perform traction or repositioning of single fracture fragments using the standard AO tubular frame (Fig. 3.2.2.1).

2. Connecting the circular frame of the Ilizarov fixator and the "rail profile" of the hybrid fixator system

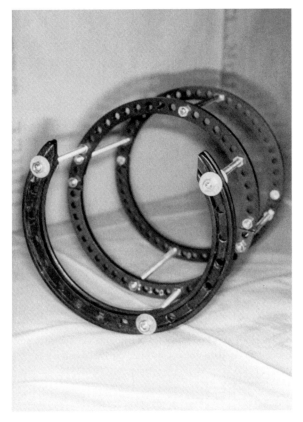

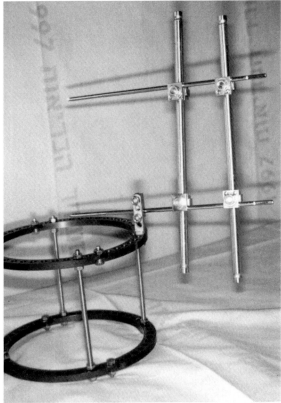

Fig. 3.2.2.2. Connecting the circular frame of the Ilizarov fixator to the "rail profile" of the hybrid fixator system by using standard washers of the Ilizarov set. *Lerner et al. Modular use of external fixation configurations for treatment of complex and severely injured limbs. Eur J Trauma 2003; 29:108–111 [77] (© Urban & Vogel. Reproduced with permission)*

Fig. 3.2.2.3. The use of some Schanz screw simultaneously in different external fixation systems (unilateral tubular external fixator and Ilizarov frame) as a simple transitional component. *Lerner et al. Modular use of external fixation configurations for treatment of complex and severely injured limbs. Eur J Trauma 2003; 29:108–111 [77] (© Urban & Vogel. Reproduced with permission)*

may be achieved by using standard washers from the Ilizarov set (Fig. 3.2.2.2).

3. Simultaneous use of the same Schanz screws in different planes of external fixation systems as a simple transitional component between frames which include these screws (Fig. 3.2.2.3).

We emphasize the use and need for only standard units of the available sets, because all the above-mentioned constructions are modular adaptations of the different frame systems and can be achieved without specially designed parts (Fig. 3.2.2.4).

Detailed preoperative planning of the surgical procedure and appropriate optimal fixation frame arrangement is mandatory to ensure success. Each external fixation frame is tailored to a concrete surgical problem and anatomical site [77]. For example, thin wires must be used in the presence of a thin or fragile bone or for

fixation of small bone fragments. In anatomical areas with a thick soft-tissue envelope, Schanz screws are recommended.

The hybrid external fixation frame combines the advantages of each system and provides sufficient closed reduction and three-plane stabilization with a minimally invasive fixation technique [77]. It allows early mobilization and reduces the risk of osteomyelitis and further tissue damage. This modular non-constrained apparatus provides the orthopedic surgeon with more options to solve complex problems common in patients suffering from high-energy limb injuries (Fig. 3.2.2.5).

This technique of combining the commonly used external fixation frames is simple and cost-efficient, and has been extensively tested under various clinical conditions (Fig. 3.2.2.6).

Standard industrially produced hybrid fixators are generally composed of one ring (half-ring or 5.8 ring)

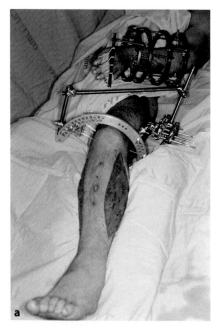

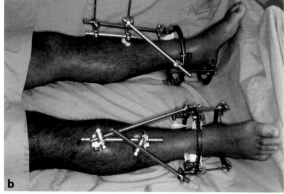

Fig. 3.2.2.4a–c. Clinical appearance of different hybrid frames using only standard units of available external fixation sets

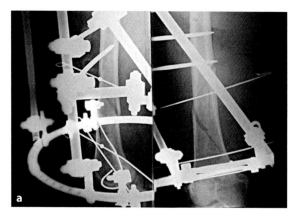

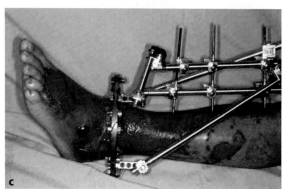

Fig. 3.2.2.5a–c. Radiological appearance of hybrid external fixation frames, containing elements from Ilizarov and AO external fixation sets. **a** Radiograph of distal femoral fracture after closed reduction and hybrid external fixation. **b–c** *see next page*

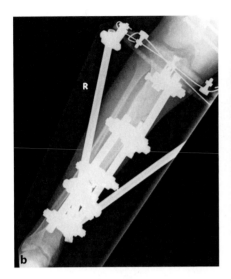
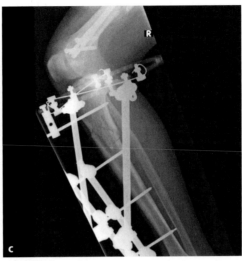

Fig. 3.2.2.5a–c. *(continued)* **b,c** Proximal tibial fracture fixed by hybrid external fixation frame

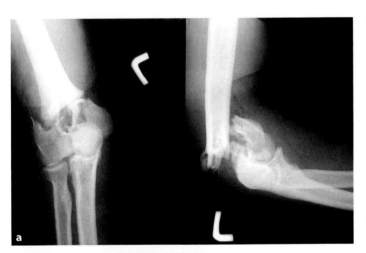
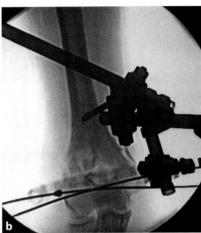

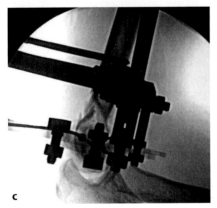

Fig. 3.2.2.6a–c. a Admission radiograph of a 25-year-old patient demonstrates displaced comminuted supra-transcondylar elbow fracture. **b,c** Anteroposterior and lateral radiographs after performing closed reduction and hybrid external fixation, using a combination of a distally placed carbon Ilizarov ring with olives thin wires and a proximally placed AO tubular frame with half-pins. *Lerner et al. Modular use of external fixation configurations for treatment of complex and severely injured limbs. Eur J Trauma 2003; 29:108–111 [77] (© Urban & Vogel. Reproduced with permission)*

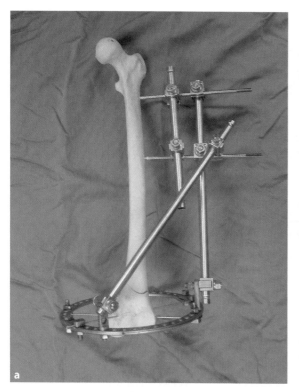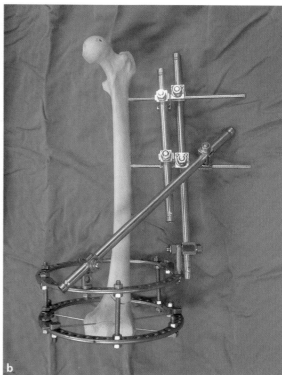

Fig. 3.2.2.7a,b. Models of the hybrid external fixation frames. **a** Standard hybrid fixation frame, **b** hybrid frame with a capacity for dynamic influence on the fracture site

placed above the metaphyseal zone, with the unilateral part above the diaphyseal zone of the injured bone. This frame achieves stable bone fixation. However, this frame has a static quality only (simple fixation frame), only fixing the position of the bone fragments, achieved by manual repositioning in the operating theater. The option of an active influence on the position of the bone fragments is absent in this frame. We recommend the use of a modified assembly of the hybrid frame; to add the capability of active reduction, one additional ring is placed between a basic (proximal or distal) ring and the unilateral unit of the hybrid fixation frame. This ring may even be "unmarried" (without any direct fixation to the bone fragments); by connecting this ring to the basic ring with threaded rods, the ability of controlled compression/distraction to the frame is gained. Threaded rods with hinges add the capacity of repairing angular deformation, and repositioning the block placed between the rings allows repair of side displacement of the fragments or malrotational deformations (Fig. 3.2.2.7).

In summary, while retaining all the positive qualities of unilateral external fixators, these hybrid assemblies have many additional unique qualities of the classic circular Ilizarov frame. This hybrid frame enables the

achievement of combined bifocal influence on the limb, producing compression/distraction forces or some correction of the deformity (circular block) on one side of the fixed segment, with static fixation on the other side (unilateral block) [77] (Fig. 3.2.2.8).

The modularity of modern external fixation sets allows building fixator assemblies suitable for each patient's specific situation. These combinations can be achieved with a minimal quantity of construction elements, avoiding the building of large, crude fixation constructions containing unnecessary components. These systems are relatively light and comfortable for patients. Moreover, they are more convenient in clinical practice. A small quantity of construction elements reduces the cost of treatment and shortens surgical time (very important in mass casualty situations). The use of modular and custom-assembled hybrid frames results in better patient compliance and a wider range of motion than is obtained with standard classic all-wire constructs.

Using combinations of different fixators enables the introduction of new properties to some fixators. For example, by adding some details to a standard Ilizarov set, it is possible to build a hinge for the functional treatment of peri-articular fractures, while continuing external fixation with a primary assembled unilateral

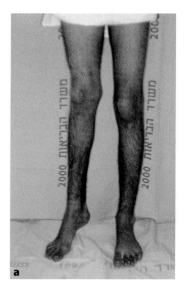

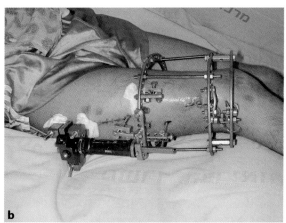

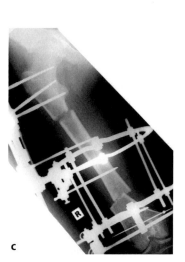

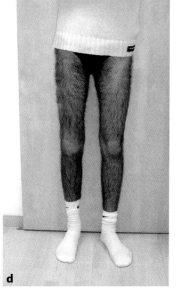

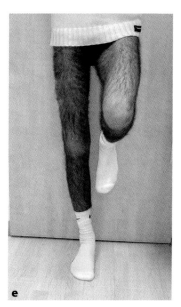

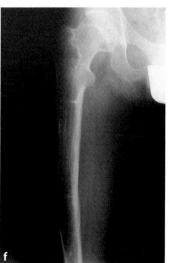

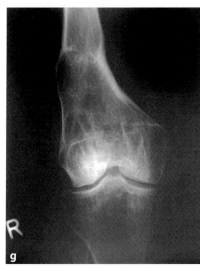

Fig. 3.2.2.8a–g. Modular hybrid external fixation frame used for treating severe combined right femoral bone deformity. **a** Clinical appearance of short right lower limb with knee valgus deformity. **b** Clinical appearance of modular combination between distally placed Ilizarov frame, and proximally placed Dinafix external fixator. **c** Radiological appearance of distal corrective femoral osteotomy, fixed using Ilizarov frame, and proximal elongation osteotomy, fixed by Dinafix external fixator. **d–g** Clinical and radiological appearance on follow-up 4 years after removal of the hybrid external frame

external fixation device. This assembly of an external fixation frame has been used successfully for the treatment of acute trauma and its consequences, and also in the management of elective orthopedic patients. Our experience in using hybrid frames allows us to recommend this method for wide use in orthopedic practice (Fig. 3.2.2.9).

3.2.3 Hinged Fixation of Peri-Articular Injuries

Severe trauma of major joints, especially the knee and the elbow, is common in modern war-related injuries [100]. These high-energy injuries are usually associated with massive soft-tissue damage and ligamental and capsular tears [139]. Reliable stabilization of the peri-articular bone fragments and early motion optimize the functional outcome of these complex injuries. This is provided by the modular circular/hybrid external fixation frame [71].

Following fixation of peri-articular fractures, the joint is examined for occult ligamentous and capsular injuries which affect anteroposterior, latero-medial and/or rotational stability. In patients with unstable knee or elbow joints, the hybrid/circular devices used for external fracture fixation from both sides of the joints are connected by hinges to achieve stability and enable immediate functional treatment (Fig. 3.2.3.1).

We recommend trans-articular hinged external fixation also for patients with massive peri-articular soft-tissue injuries associated with high-energy fractures. This method allows temporary bridging of the injured joint, as well as the performance of controlled passive movement (very important in the treatment of multiply injured or unconscious patients, in treating articular stiffness and in complex injuries, including burns). Equally, passive movement is afforded to patients with severe neuromuscular damage who are temporarily unable to perform active motion of the injured joints (Fig. 3.2.3.2).

The adjustment of one additional ring (or 5/8 ring) from the opposite side of the joint is a widely used tool in the treatment of peri-articular fractures, using ligamentotaxis for the closed reduction of the bone fragments. In some patients, the presence of a short (or comminuted) peri-articular bone fragment mandates that this additional trans-articular fixation should be preserved for a supplemental period of 3–4 weeks of rigid fixation, and only then demounted, proceeding to delayed joint mobilization.

At the end of such an operative procedure, some articular distraction in the frame must be preserved to avoid compression and subsequent displacement of the bone fragments. Incidentally, during the period of rigid trans-articular fixation, it is possible to perform not only active and passive motions in the adjacent non-fixed joints but also axial loading of the injured

limb (weight-bearing in patients with lower limb injuries).

When a sufficient level of fracture fixation is not achieved (multi-fragmental fractures, extremely short peri-articular fragment), and also in the presence of severe damage to the articular capsule and ligaments, it is necessary to institute prolonged trans-articular dynamic fixation. For this purpose, after finishing definitive reduction and fixation of the fracture, the threaded rods of the trans-articular fixation device are changed to hinged rods placed in the axis of articular motions. In patients with significant damage to the peri-articular soft tissues, the hinge motion can be temporarily blocked by tightening the hinge nut on its axis of motion and/or by applying a temporary rigid crossbar. This crossbar will be demounted after healing of the soft-tissue wound for mobilization of the previously locked joint. The mechanical proprieties of such a modular external fixation frame allow, if needed, the temporary limitation of the range of motion according to the level of the achieved stability, condition of the wound, and tendo-muscular and neuro-vascular damage.

The most important step in assembling the trans-articular hinged fixation is the proper placing of the axis for articular motion. A mistake in the setting of the hinge axis can create displacing forces, causing damage to the articular cartilage created by over-compression or damage to the ligamentary complex by over-distraction. In addition to taking account of anatomical landmarks, as recommended in appropriate publications, we do not primarily attach the hinge firmly to the corresponding ring, but observe the hinge during articular motions. Declination of the hinge from the ring during these articular motions indicates an incorrect selection of the rotation axis of the joint. This dynamic test must be repeated after changing the location of the hinge. A lack of displacement of the hinge during articular motions is a good indicator for the accurate selection of the axis of motion. Only then can the hinges be firmly fixed to the corresponding proximal and distal rings. This procedure must be repeated from the opposite side of the trans-fixed joint.

It is also possible to perform some small distraction of the joints on the hinges in order to avoid compression of the joint cartilage and intra-articular bone fragments and subsequent displacement of the fractures during further articular mobilization. This is assessed as a joint space of 1–2 mm on the check radiograph. But it is important to avoid articular over-distraction resulting in pain, contractures, and problems in the capsular and ligamentous healing.

Contrary to some existing configurations of external articular hinged fixation frames, we do not use articular axial wires. This is in agreement with Nechaev et al. [99] who stated that there are difficulties and complications associated with the insertion of an axial wire: damage

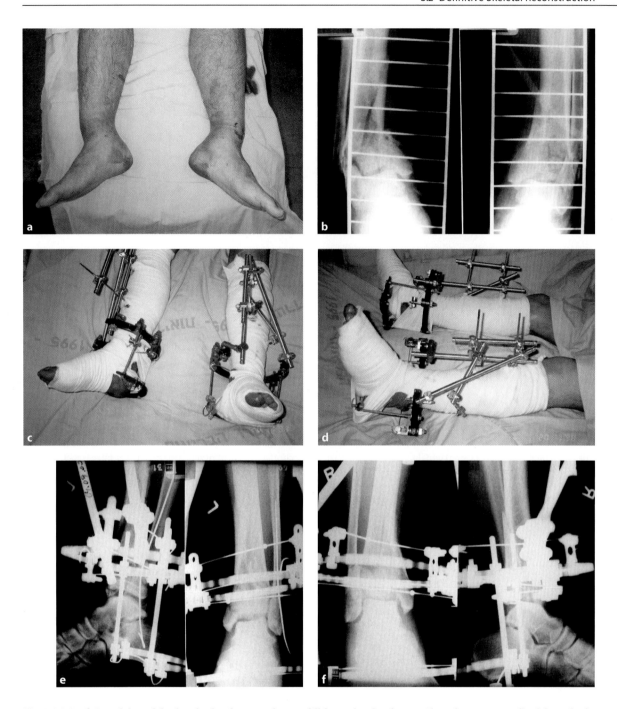

Fig. 3.2.2.9a–f. Open bilateral displaced pylon fractures due to a fall from a height of 6 m. **a** Clinical appearance of both lower limbs on admission. **b** Radiographs of comminuted displaced bilateral pylon fractures on admission. **c–f** Clinical and radiological appearance after closed reduction and external fixation with hybrid frames

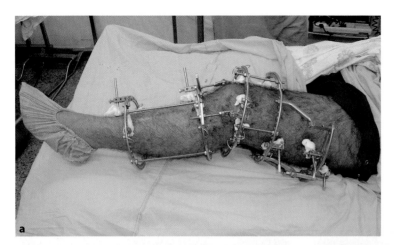

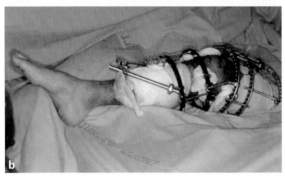

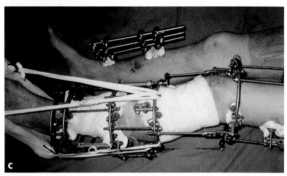

Fig. 3.2.3.1a–c. Hinged Ilizarov external fixation frames used for functional treatment of severe peri-articular knee fractures

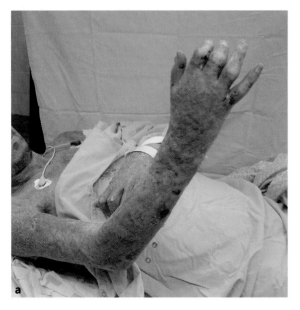

Fig. 3.2.3.2a–e. A 37-year-old male suffering from full-thickness circular burns to his right upper extremity caused by an open fire. The Ilizarov device was used to handle post-burn contracture. **a** Clinical pre-operative appearance of the right upper limb. Note severe extensive scaring and 60° post-burn elbow contracture. **b–e** *see next page*

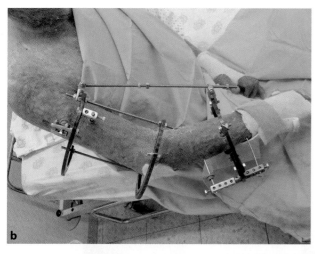
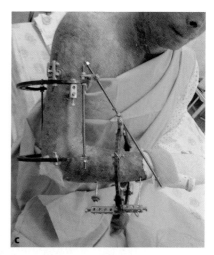
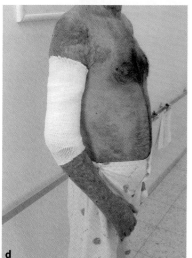
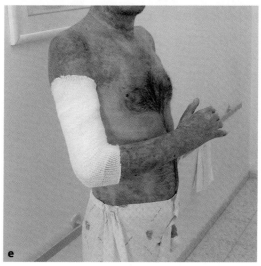

Fig. 3.2.3.2a–e. *(continued)* **b,c** Clinical appearance of passive elbow mobilization using Ilizarov external fixation frame with trans-articular placed threaded rod. **d,e** Follow-up after 6 months. Note active elbow motions between 40° and 100°

to the articular cartilage of the joint, damage to nearby nerves (ulnar nerve damage by insertion of the thin wire through the condylar zone of the humeral bone), and trans-fixation of the articular capsule of the knee joint that can lead to a painful syndrome and restriction of knee motions. Therefore, we justify the use of an axial articular wire only if it is absolutely necessary for the mechanical fixation of intra- or peri-articular bone fragments.

Range of movement exercises are recommended as tolerated, avoiding pain, relating to muscular spasm and blockage of the motions. Remember that restoring articular motions requires much effort and time. Moreover, trans-fixation of soft tissues in the external fixation frame leads to some restriction of movement in the adjacent joints which will remain until the transfixing elements are removed.

The necessity for trans-articular fixation recedes during the consolidation and maturation of the fracture callus. At that time, the ring on the opposite site of the joint and hinges can be dismounted. External fixation of the fracture itself is continued until fracture consolidation is sufficient for definitive reassembly of the fixation frame (Fig. 3.2.3.3).

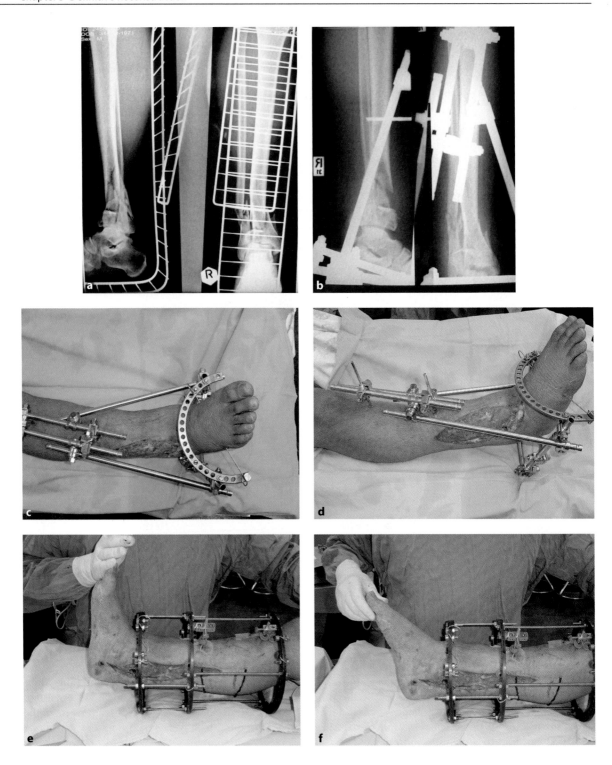

Fig. 3.2.3.3a–w. A 27-year-old male suffering from open Gustilo–Anderson type IIIA right pylon fracture with severe bone comminution due to road traffic accident. Fasciotomy was performed during primary debridement due to acute compartment syndrome.
a Radiograph at time of injury. Note severe bone comminuting and displacement of distal tibial bone fragments. **b** Radiograph after
primary stabilization of the fracture, including temporary ankle joint bridging, using hybrid external fixation. **c,d** Clinical appearance of the right lower limb fixed with a hybrid frame. Note good post-fasciotomy wound coverage after skin grafting procedure.
e,f Conversion of hybrid fixator to Ilizarov circular frame is performed. Clinical appearance of intra-operative passive ankle motions
on the operating table. **g–w** *see next pages*

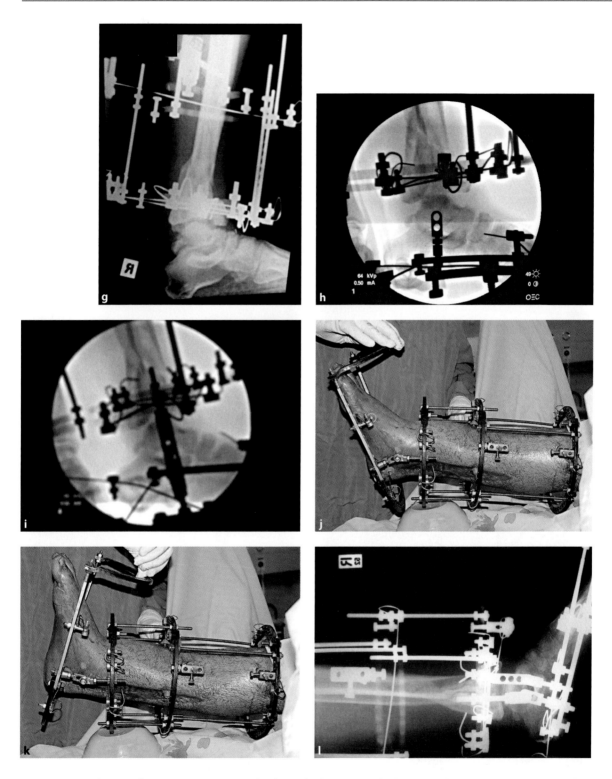

Fig. 3.2.3.3a–w. *(continued)* **g** Intra-operative control radiographs demonstrate displacement of the intra-articular anterior tibial bone fragment. **h,i** Decision to perform trans-ankle dynamic stabilization using additional foot ring was made. Intra-operative radiographs demonstrate the process of choosing the right place for hinges above the center of the talar dome (axis motion of ankle). **j,k** Clinical photos of controlled passive tibio-talar motions in the trans-ankle stabilization frame. **l** Radiographs demonstrate additional fixation of anterior bone fragment using short olive wire as pusher. **m–w** *see next pages*

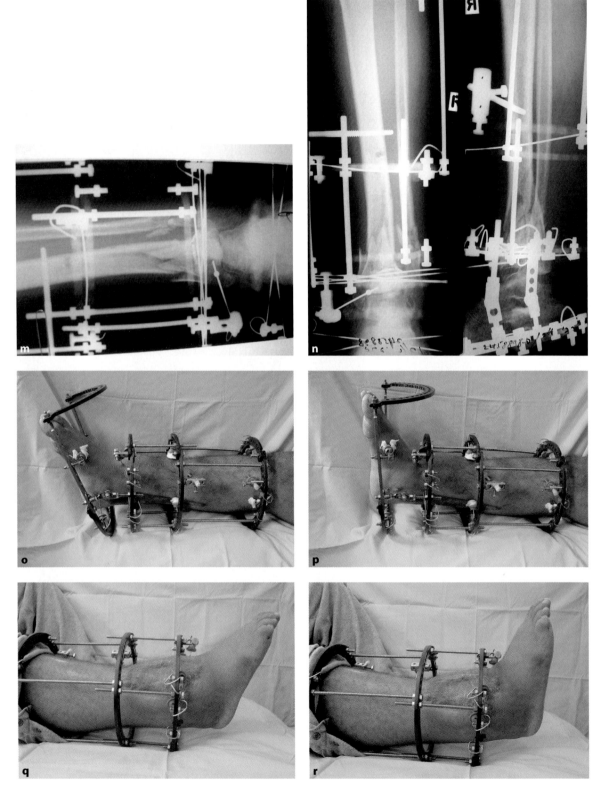

Fig. 3.2.3.3a–w. *(continued)* **m** Radiographs demonstrate additional fixation of anterior bone fragment using short olive wire as pusher. **n** Radiograph 3 months after conversion to Ilizarov fixation frame demonstrates signs of the bone consolidation, **o,p** Clinical appearance of active motions in the post-operative period. **q,r** Foot ring was removed after 2 months of dynamic trans-ankle fixation. Clinical appearance of active ankle mobilization during continued fracture fixation in circular tibial frame. **s–w** *see next page*

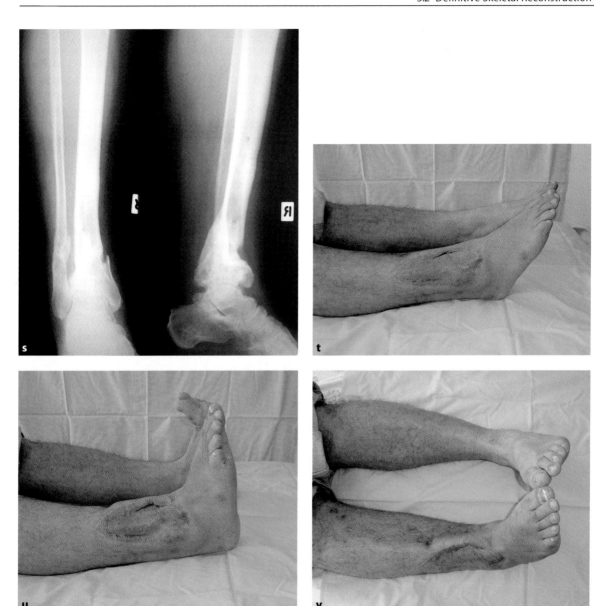

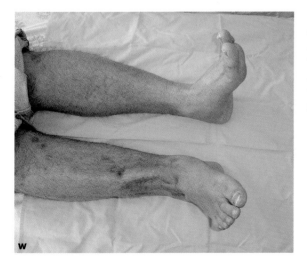

Fig. 3.2.3.3a–w. *(continued)* **s** After another month of external fixation, the Ilizarov frame was removed. Radiographs 1 year after removing the Ilizarov frame demonstrate bone healing of the fracture in good alignment with preservation of the articular surface. **t–w** Clinical photos at follow-up 1 year after removing the Ilizarov frame. Note good range of active motions in the ankle and subtalar joints

3.2.4 Peculiarity of Elbow Joint Reconstruction: Methods of Isolated Hybrid External Fixation of Humeral, Ulnar, and Radial Bones

According to Bilic et al. [8], the elbow is the most susceptible joint of the upper limb to war injury.

The elbow joint has a poor potential for good function after high-energy injuries, even after anatomic realignment. The fractures are unstable, may have an intra-articular component, and present a challenging problem. According to Graham and Fitzgerald [41], the destroyed elbow is usually characterized by a global injury to bone and soft tissue. Penetrating projectile high-energy injuries to upper limbs are commonly encountered with various neurovascular injuries and compartment syndrome. According to Wilson [144], reconstruction of elbow fractures is difficult because of the complex anatomy and desire to maintain postoperative motion. He wrote: "Limited attempts of internal fixation and reconstruction may fail because of the high concentration of force; treatment concepts include restoration of the articular segment, rigid fixation to allow early ROM, and balance of soft tissue repair for stability." Fracture type and degree of comminuting and soft-tissue injury influence the type of fixation required. Ilizarov external fixation requires minimal soft-tissue dissection while still allowing stable fixation, functional alignment, and early commencement of movement of the elbow and forearm. The continuous implementation of active exercises to enhance the range of elbow movements reduces the likelihood of severe capsular contractures. It is minimally invasive and thus allows soft-tissue protection, reducing the potential for infection.

Circular external fixation of upper limb fractures, especially forearm fractures resulting from gunshot wounds and blast injuries, has not received particular attention in the literature. Primary stabilization in patients suffering from severe high-energy peri-articular fractures is performed according to the aforesaid principles of primary fixation of fractures. However, this specific anatomical locality of fracture necessitates some special tricks for fixation. The complex neurovascular topography dictates the strict abidance of safe zones during insertion of thin wires and half-pins to the bone. As a rule, a pair of half-pins into each side of the fracture is enough for the primary fixation of bone fragments. Distal humeral fractures and severe intra-articular elbow fractures need temporary articular bridging. Proximal half-pins introduced into the bone at the level of the proximal and mid-third of the humeral bone, and the application of proximal pins of the external fixator through the humeral head are needed in extended comminuted humeral shaft fractures [24]. A distal half-pin should be introduced at the level of the proximal third of the ulnar bone. The relatively small diameter of the ulnar bone in the mid-third demands the use of small-diameter half-

pins to prevent iatrogenic fractures. Primary fixation at the forearm level in patients with comminuting of the proximal ulnar bone is executed by inserting half-pins to the distal radial bone. Such a frame provides relatively lesser stability of fixation due to the comparatively long area of the injured segment between the proximal and distal pairs of half-pins. Therefore, these configurations demand earlier conversion to a final fixation frame. Additional fixation of the forearm bones using mini-external fixation sets is used in treating patients with multiple comminuted fractures.

We usually use half-pins in performing conversion of the primary assembled tubular external fixator to the final circular frame, inserted to the humeral bone during primary fixation (with accurate localization, good stability in the bone, and in the absence of local soft-tissue problems). It is necessary to insert a third half-pin or thin wire in some patients to increase the stability of fracture fixation. External fixation of the distal humeral fragment is a technically difficult procedure. For this purpose, we prefer to use two thin olive wires inserted through the internal and external humeral epicondyles. An additional half-pin, located more proximally and inserted through the postero-lateral bone surface, will provide sufficient stability in fixation of the distal bone fragment. Over-distraction and diastases between bone fragments must be avoided in the finishing touches of fracture fixation, because this can extend the time of external fixation in the frame significantly. The likelihood of non-union is also increased. In contrast, a relative shortening of the healed humeral bone will not affect future upper limb function. Using commercially available hinged elbow external fixators is technically demanding [132]. The most critical step is the correct placement of the axial pin. Care must be taken to protect the ulnar nerve during insertion of the axial pin. In contrast, the Ilizarov external fixator provides for mounting a hinged frame without requiring a precisely inserted and potentially dangerous axial wire (Fig. 3.2.4.1).

Utilizing only a small number of parts from the standard Ilizarov set, it is possible in some cases to assemble a hinge for a unilateral tubular external fixator, one that allows preserving stability of fixation and simultaneous early mobilization of the fixed joint (Fig. 3.2.4.2).

In cases of forearm injuries, it is very important to preserve pronation/supination motions during the period of external fixation. According to Wilson [144], non-union and malunion of the forearm bones are more likely to occur than synostosis and, therefore, rotational motions must be preserved during the prolonged period of treatment of severe high-energy trauma to the forearm bones. This requirement can be guaranteed only by utilizing a method of separate bone fixation for each of the forearm bones. To solve this technical problem, we propose: fixation of the forearm bones in a pair of *separate* unilateral frames, circular frames, or hybrid fixators. We prefer separate fixation of forearm bones in

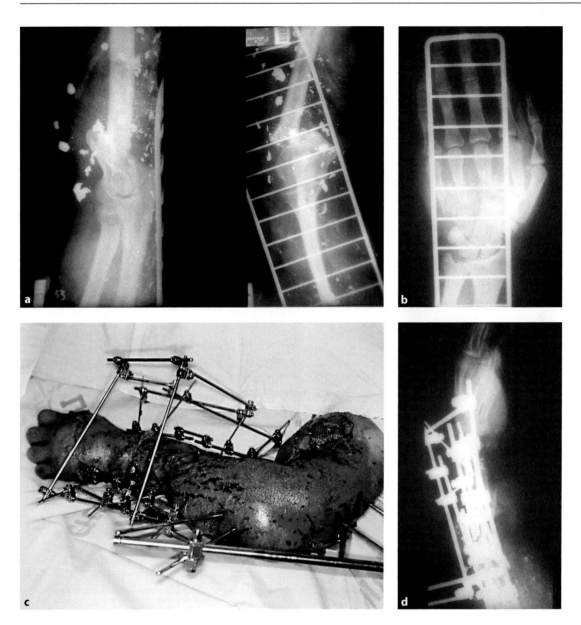

Fig. 3.2.4.1a–q. A 20-year-old male who suffered an anti-tank rocket blast injury to the left upper limb was admitted to our hospital 1 h after trauma, with open multi-comminuted fractures of left humerus, ulna and radius Gustilo–Anderson IIIB, multiple metacarpal fractures, and a penetrating chest injury. After stabilization of the general condition, including tracheostomy and thoracotomy, primary debridement and external stabilization of the left upper limb using AO and Mini-AO external fixation frames with temporary elbow bridging was performed. **a,b** Radiographs of left upper limb on admission demonstrate multiple fractures and presence of multiple metal foreign bodies. **c** Clinical appearance of the left upper limb after primary external fixation and elbow bridging. **d** Radiograph after primary external fixation. **e–q** *see next page*

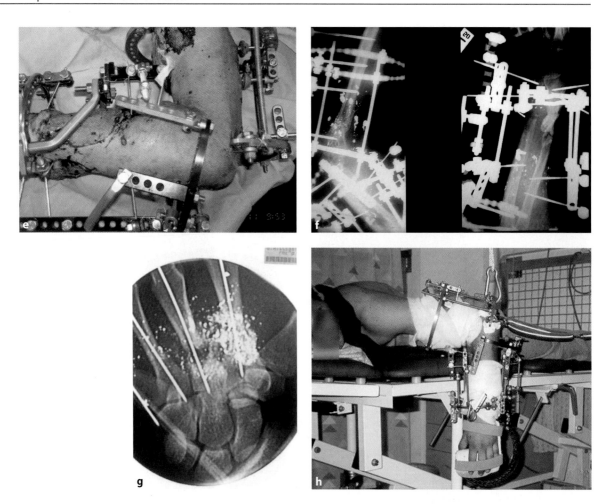

Fig. 3.2.4.1a–q. *(continued)* **e** Seven days later, conversion of tubular fixation to hybrid external fixation frames was performed. Skin grafts were used to close the granulating soft tissues. The clinical appearance of the upper limb shows the isolated hybrid fixation of humeral, ulnar and radial bones. Note the temporary communication between ulnar and radial external fixation frames using a threaded rod for early passive pronation/supination motions due to severe traumatic soft-tissue damage. **f,g** Radiological appearance after closed reduction and external fixation of humeral, ulnar and radial factures. The metacarpal fractures are fixed using intramedullary placed thin wires. Note presence of multiple metallic foreign bodies in tissues of the upper limb. **h** Passive and active mobilization was initiated in the early post-operative period. Clinical photo shows functional treatment in the physiotherapy department. **i–q** *see next page*

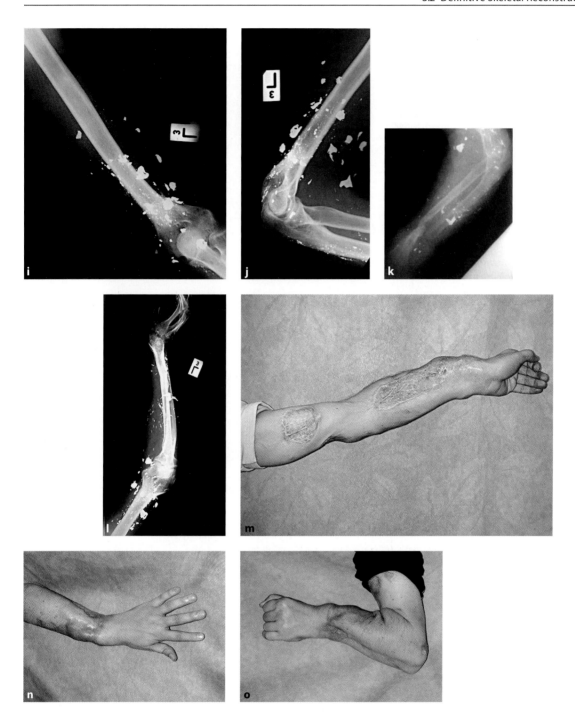

Fig. 3.2.4.1a–q. *(continued)* **i–l** Hybrid external fixation frames were removed after 5 months of external fixation. Radiological examination 1 year after removing the fixation frames demonstrates bone consolidation in good alignment. Note multiple foreign bodies in the tissues. **m–o** Clinical appearance on follow-up 1 year after removing hybrid fixation frames. Note functional range of active elbow flexion and extension, forearm pronation and supination, and hand motions. **p–q** *see next page*

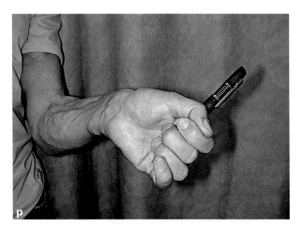

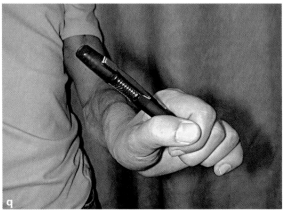

Fig. 3.2.4.1a–q. *(continued)* **p–q** Clinical appearance on follow-up 1 year after removing hybrid fixation frames. Note functional range of active elbow flexion and extension, forearm pronation and supination, and hand motions

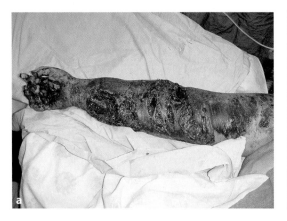

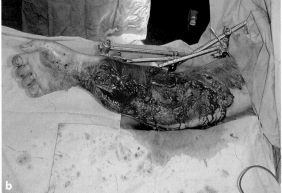

Fig. 3.2.4.2a–k. A 38-year-old female with open right elbow dislocation, extensive soft-tissue damage and skin loss on arm and forearm. Immediate debridement and reduction of the elbow dislocation was performed. A trans-elbow unilateral external fixation frame was used postoperatively to keep the elbow joint in a position of reduction. **a** Clinical appearance of the right upper limb on admission illustrates extensive soft-tissue damage. **b** Clinical appearance after primary external fixation and temporary elbow bridging. **c–k** *see next page*

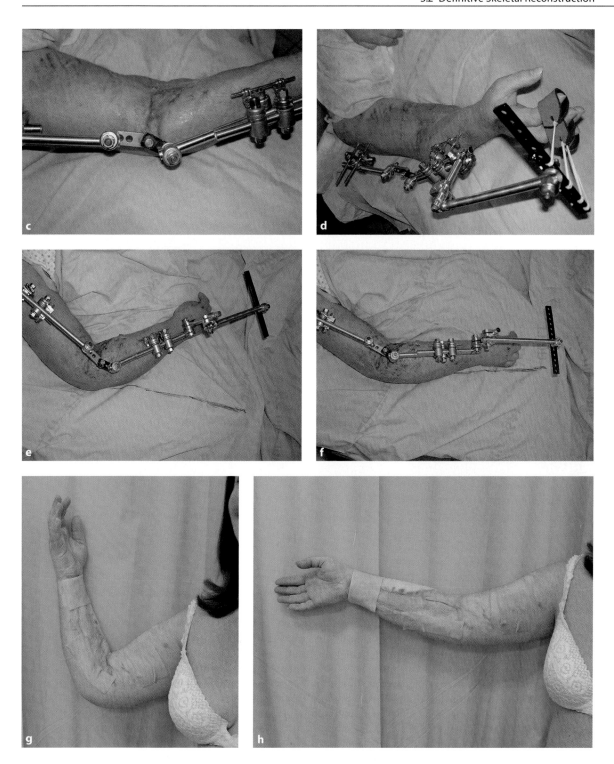

Fig. 3.2.4.2a–k. *(continued)* **c** Mobile hinge composed of simple elements from the Ilizarov set was inserted into the external fixation frame at the level of the elbow rotation center to allow early functional treatment during period of external fixation. Clinical photo shows the mobile elbow hinge. **d** Clinical appearance of post-traumatic radial nerve palsy; dynamic finger splinting during external fixation period. **e,f** Early passive and active elbow motions were initiated from the first postoperative day. Clinical photos demonstrates ROM after 2 weeks of mobilization. **g–h** External fixation frame was removed after 6 weeks. Clinical appearance on follow-up 1 year after injury. Note functional range of active elbow flexion and extension, forearm pronation and supination. **i–k** *see next page*

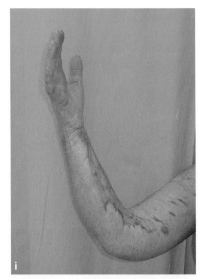

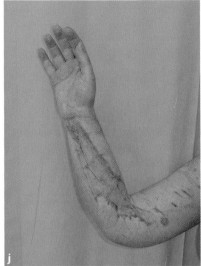

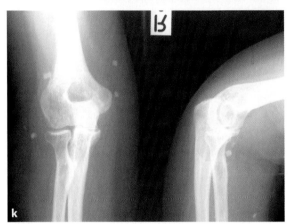

Fig. 3.2.4.2a–k. *(continued)* **i–j** External fixation frame was removed after 6 weeks. Clinical appearance on follow-up 1 year after injury. Note functional range of active elbow flexion and extension, forearm pronation and supination. **k** Radiological examination at follow-up 1 year after injury reveals multiple foreign bodies (glass splinters) in peri-articular soft tissues

two hybrid external fixation frames [74, 78]. The ring (or half-ring) is placed above the distal fragment of the radius and attached to the bone using thin wires and half-pins. The unilateral part of this fixator is disposed over the proximal radial fragment and fixed to the bone using two or three small-diameter half-pins.

We perform the stabilization of the ulnar bone in the reverse order: a half-ring above the proximal bone fragment (fixed using thin wires and half-pins) with the unilateral part of the frame attached to the distal bone fragment using small-diameter half-pins. This method of fixation of forearm bones allows rotational motions during the period of external skeletal fixation. Connection between these separate hybrid external fixators using one threaded rod with nuts allows passive rotational motions in patients, in whom the possibility of active motion is temporarily lost due to extensive neuromuscular damage. Generally, severe complex fractures of both forearm bones dictate an individual approach

according to each specific clinical situation. A modular fixation frame must be arranged according to the fracture's configuration and soft-tissue condition. An opposite order of preoperative planning, with "heroic" attempts to squeeze the severe complex fracture to the "Procrust's bed" of the standard available fixation frame must be discarded. Active and assisted passive motions should be initiated on the second postoperative day for most patients (Fig. 3.2.4.3).

To treat patients with extensive multi-comminuted fractures of the humeral bone, it is possible to perform closed reduction and sufficient fixation in the acceptable alignment using the hybrid external fixation frame as "a mobile skeletal traction device" with a minimal number of inserted thin wires and half-pins. Two or three half-pins are inserted to the proximal main fragment of the humeral bone. Only one distally placed thin wire, introduced through the olecranon in the coronal direction, is sufficient to allow closed reduction of the

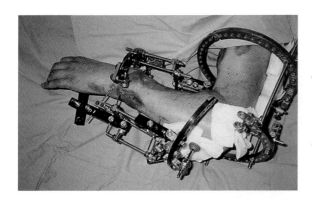

Fig. 3.2.4.3. Isolated external fixation of humeral, ulnar and radial bones using hybrid external fixation frames

bone fragments, using the method of ligamentotaxis. Moreover, this provides early functional mobilization of the elbow joint (Fig. 3.2.4.4).

The rich blood circulation in the upper limb provides a relatively high potential of regeneration and, in the absence of weight-bearing loading, allows the possibility of functional restoration, even in patients with very severe injuries. According to the literature, a primary neurological deficit after gunshot wounds to the upper limb resolves in time in 70% of patients without any specific intervention [82]. Therefore, indications for primary amputations even after devastating injuries to upper limbs must be severely restricted (Fig. 3.2.4.5).

3.2.5 Bilateral Lower Limb Injuries

Bilateral lower limb injuries are often encountered in severe road traffic accidents (RTA) or war injuries. They severely restrict the patient's mobility, causing lengthy periods of bed-rest [73]. When both legs are severely injured, the patient can only mobilize him or herself early if the fracture fixation method successfully provides full weight-bearing of at least one of the injured limbs (Fig. 3.2.5.1).

Modern methods of internal fixation, especially the use of massive intramedullary nails with locking, allow functional weight-bearing in diaphyseal fractures. However, in cases in which the use of internal fixation devices carries a great risk of severe complications and in treating patients suffering from severe bone loss and those with severe comminuted, especially intra-articular fractures, the use of intramedullary nailing is precluded. The bed-rest period may be prolonged up to half a year or even more. Such a long period of bed-rest can result in both physical and psychological complications. The degree of stability of fixation in the circular Ilizarov frame is sufficient to allow full weight-bear-

ing on the injured limb even in the presence of major bone loss [70]. Stable external fixation of at least one of the limbs in the Ilizarov frame allows mobilization and early weight-bearing on this limb with crutches. This affords a good basis for functional treatment of the injured contralateral leg (Fig. 3.2.5.2, Fig. 3.2.5.3, Fig. 3.2.5.4, Fig. 3.2.5.5).

3.2.6 Lower Limb Salvage Where Contralateral Amputation is Present

Bilateral injury to the lower extremities that results in amputation of one leg and limb salvage surgery on the other is a situation of unusual complexity and one that requires surgeons to use considerable foresight in determining treatment strategies. The Ilizarov external fixation device is indicated in cases of limb salvage where contralateral amputation is present, as it fulfills the criteria for early amputee rehabilitation while simultaneously achieving cyclic loading that facilitates fracture healing. The treatment strategy for patients with severe bilateral lower limb injuries merits in-depth analysis since unilateral limb loss extensively influences "the reconstruction ladder" of the contralateral limb. The main advantage of this method is that each limb can be managed by an "isolated injury approach" basis, thereby preventing cross-interference in treatment. The patient's capability to bear full weight on the limb, fixed using a circular external fixation device, allows the unimpeded independent and concomitant adjustment of the prosthesis [73] (Fig. 3.2.6.1, Fig. 3.2.6.2, Fig. 3.2.6.3).

3.2.7 Primary Arthrodesis After High-Energy Injuries

An attempt at anatomical restoration of the articular surface and stable fixation of the bone fragments must be performed in the treatment of patients suffering from intra-articular fractures. After using minimal internal fixation methods, open reduction with additional fixation in an external frame, if needed, must be performed in the treatment of patients in which an attempt at closed reduction was unsuccessful. When the articular surface has disintegrated, the external fixator maintains length before arthrodesis, arthroplasty, or articular grafting [144]. Sometimes, however, severe and extensive articular and peri-articular destruction makes surgical salvage impossible. Arthrodesis is a widely accepted surgical salvage procedure for various severe joint pathologies. Arthrodesis as an alternative to limb amputation has many functional and psychological benefits. Primary arthrodesis has been advocated as a treatment for severe intra-articular fractures with severe tissue loss [52]. A multitude of different methods

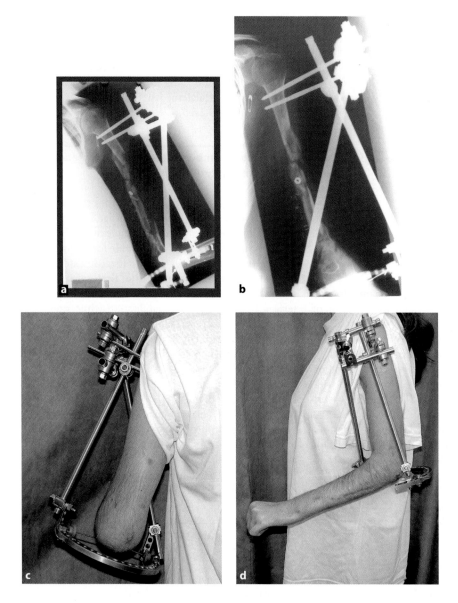

Fig. 3.2.4.4a–o. A 19-year-old female suffering from a blast injury to left upper limb in a suicide bus blast was admitted with open multi-comminuted fracture of left humerus Gustilo–Anderson type IIIA. Primary treatment included debridement and external stabilization of the left upper limb using a hybrid external fixation frame. Proximal half-pins were inserted into the proximal humeral bone but, due to severe comminution of the midshaft and distal humerus, a distal thin wire was inserted through the olecranon, with trans-elbow assembly of the fixation frame. Closed reduction of the bone fragments using the ligamentotaxis technique was performed. **a,b** Radiographs of the right upper limb after hybrid external fixation. Note multi-comminuted humeral fracture and presence of foreign body – metallic nut – in the fracture zone. **c–d** Clinical appearance of the left upper limb fixed by hybrid trans-elbow frame. Note active elbow motions during surgical stabilization. **e–o** *see next page*

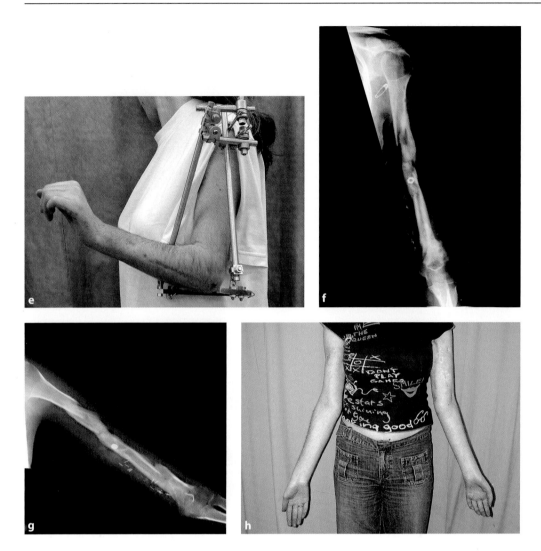

Fig. 3.2.4.4a–o. *(continued)* **e** Clinical appearance of the left upper limb fixed by hybrid trans-elbow frame. Note active elbow motions during surgical stabilization. **f,g** Hybrid fixation frame was removed after 5 months of external fixation. Radiological examination after removing the fixation frame demonstrates bone consolidation in good alignment. **h** Clinical appearance on follow-up 2 years after removing the hybrid fixation frame. Note full range of active shoulder, elbow, and hand motions. **i–k** *see next page*

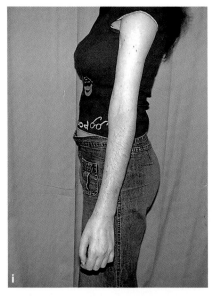

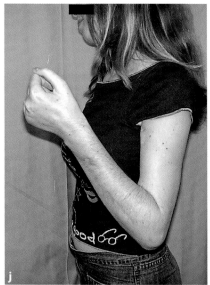

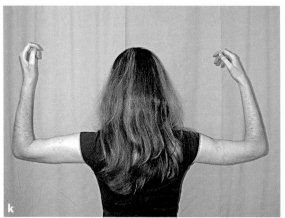

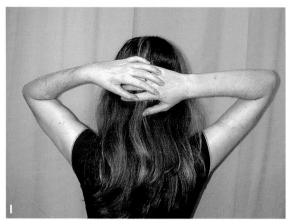

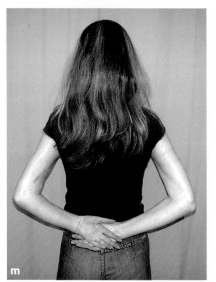

Fig. 3.2.4.4a–o. *(continued)* **i–m** Clinical appearance on follow-up 2 years after removing the hybrid fixation frame. Note full range of active shoulder, elbow, and hand motions. **n–o** *see next page*

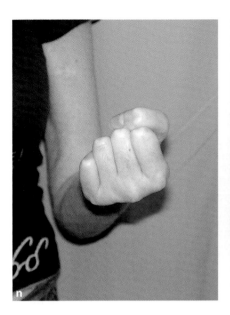
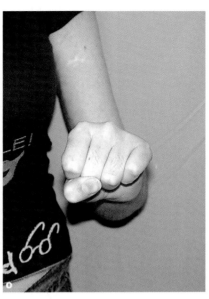

Fig. 3.2.4.4a–o. *(continued)* **n–o** Clinical appearance on follow-up 2 years after removing the hybrid fixation frame. Note full range of active shoulder, elbow, and hand motions

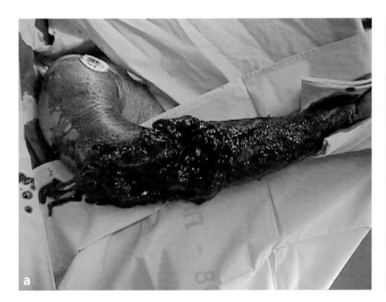
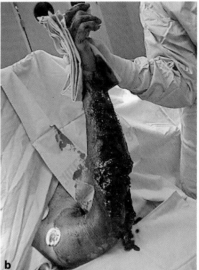

Fig. 3.2.4.5a–x. A 33-year-old male suffering from a blast injury caused by an anti-tank rocket to the right upper limb. **a,b** Clinical appearance on admission of severely injured right upper limb with deep extended skin and soft-tissue loss and burn injury to the elbow region and forearm. **c–x** *see next page*

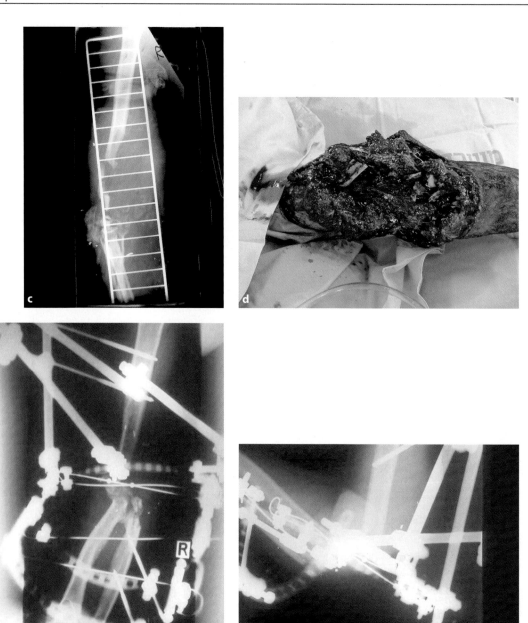

Fig. 3.2.4.5a–x. *(continued)* **c** Radiological examination on admission demonstrates destroyed elbow joint and fractures of humeral, ulnal, and radial bones. Note bone loss of the distal humerus, severe comminuting of proximal ulnal and radial bones. **d** Clinical appearance after performing copious irrigation of the wound. **e–f** Primary treatment included radical debridement of wounds with acute shortening of the injured upper limb and external stabilization using modular hinged hybrid external fixator. Postoperative radiographs demonstrate radio-humeral re-alignment and external fixation. Early passive mobilization of the elbow was started on the 3rd postoperative day. Note radiological signs of motions on the lateral radiographs. **g–x** *see next page*

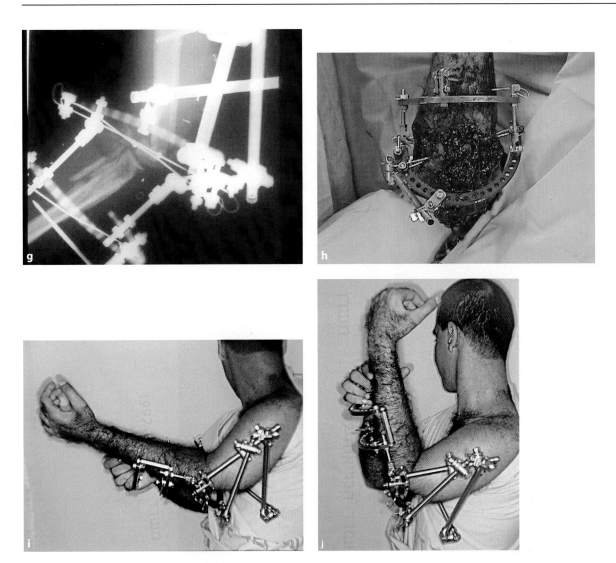

Fig. 3.2.4.5a–x. *(continued)* **g** Primary treatment included radical debridement of wounds with acute shortening of the injured upper limb and external stabilization using modular hinged hybrid external fixator. Postoperative radiographs demonstrate radio-humeral re-alignment and external fixation. Early passive mobilization of the elbow was started on the 3rd postoperative day. Note radiological signs of motions on the lateral radiographs. **h** Postoperative posterior view of the injured upper limb. Note that the fracture site is closed, due to acute upper limb shortening. **i,j** Clinical appearance of passive elbow motions during period of external fixation. **k–x** *see next page*

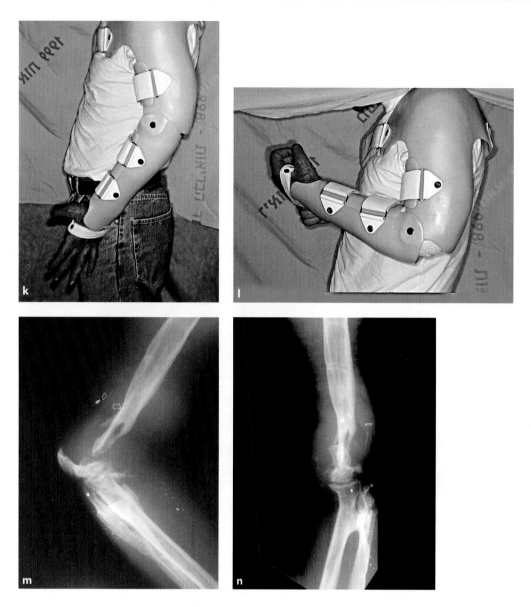

Fig. 3.2.4.5a–x. k,l Hybrid Ilizarov frame was removed after 3 months of external fixation. Additional fixation of the upper limb using hinged plastic brace was continued for another 6 months. Clinical appearance of active elbow motions with hinged stabilization in the plastic brace. **m,n** Radiological examination on follow-up 2 years after removing Ilizarov external fixation frame. Note radiological appearance of the elbow pseudo-arthrosis. **o–x** *see next page*

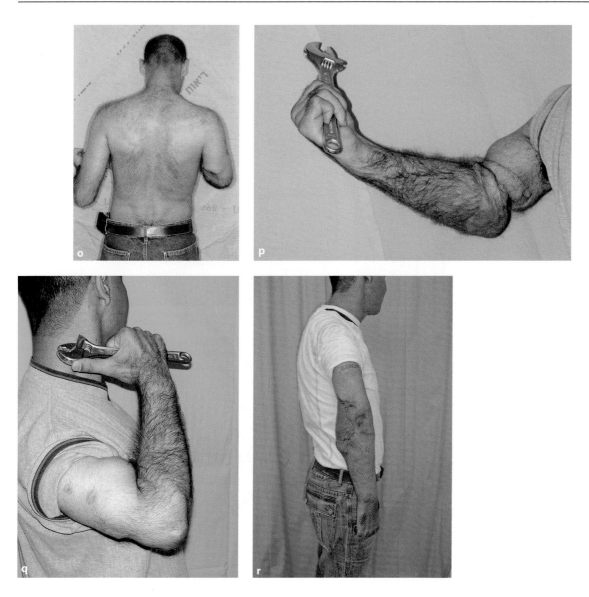

Fig. 3.2.4.5a–x. o–r Clinical appearance on follow-up 2 years after removing the Ilizarov fixation frame. Note full range of active elbow motions. Right upper limb is highly functional (elbow, wrist and fingers motions, load lifting, wringing), even with unstable elbow pseudo-arthrosis. **s–x** *see next page*

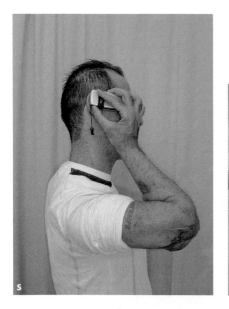

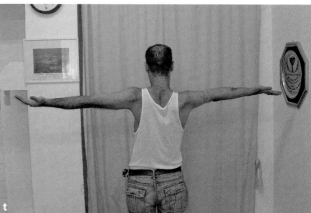

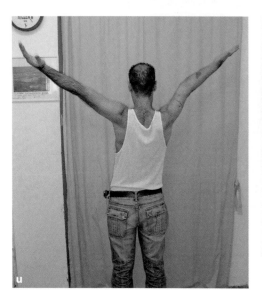

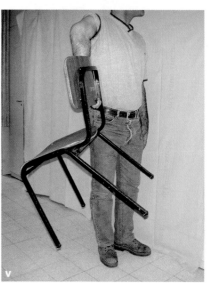

Fig. 3.2.4.5a–x. *(continued)* **s–v** Clinical appearance on follow-up 2 years after removing the Ilizarov fixation frame. Note full range of active elbow motions. Right upper limb is highly functional (elbow, wrist and fingers motions, load lifting, wringing), even with unstable elbow pseudo-arthrosis. **w–x** *see next page*

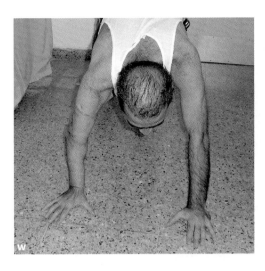
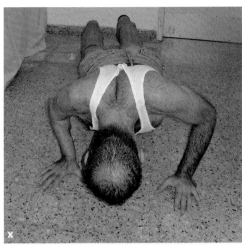

Fig. 3.2.4.5a–x. *(continued)* **w–x** Clinical appearance on follow-up 2 years after removing the Ilizarov fixation frame. Note full range of active elbow motions. Right upper limb is highly functional (elbow, wrist and fingers motions, load lifting, wringing), even with unstable elbow pseudo-arthrosis

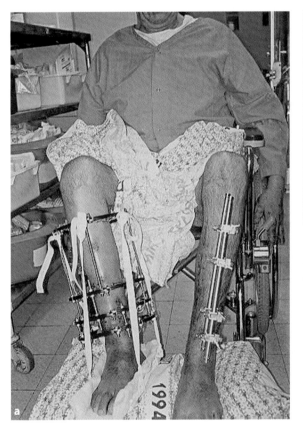

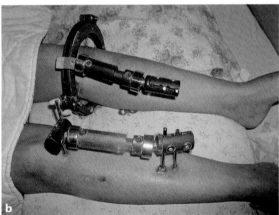

Fig. 3.2.5.1a–c. Clinical appearance of different types of external fixation devices, used for primary stabilization in treating patients with severe bilateral lower limb injuries

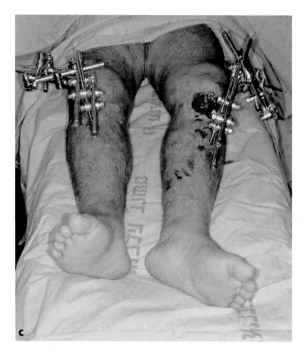

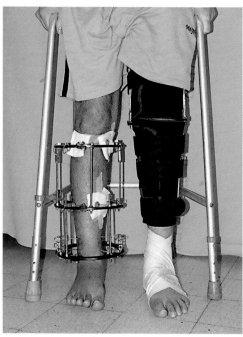

Fig. 3.2.5.1a–c. Clinical appearance of different types of external fixation devices, used for primary stabilization in treating patients with severe bilateral lower limb injuries

Fig. 3.2.5.2. Clinical appearance of early weight-bearing after severe bilateral lower limb injury: comminuted distal left tibial fracture, fixed by Ilizarov frame, and totally unstable left knee joint fixed by knee brace

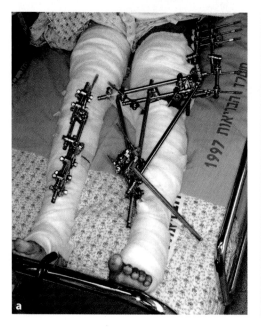

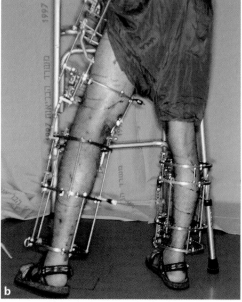

Fig. 3.2.5.3a–f. A 19-year-old male with bilateral comminuted tibial fractures and left femoral fractures due to blast mine injury. **a** Clinical appearance of the primary stabilization using tubular external fixation frames with temporary left knee bridging. **b** Seven days later, conversion from tubular frames to circular Ilizarov devices was performed with freeing of left knee joint (hinges allow communication between left tibial and femoral external fixation frames). Clinical photos demonstrate early weight-bearing and walking during external fixation in the Ilizarov frames. **c–f** *see next page*

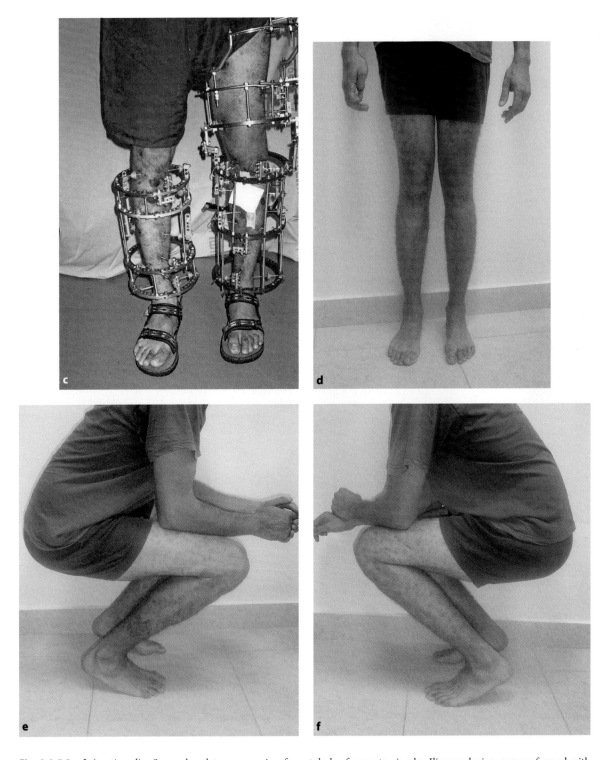

Fig. 3.2.5.3a–f. *(continued)* **c** Seven days later, conversion from tubular frames to circular Ilizarov devices was performed with freeing of left knee joint (hinges allow communication between left tibial and femoral external fixation frames). Clinical photos demonstrate early weight-bearing and walking during external fixation in the Ilizarov frames. **d–f** Follow up 8 years latter. Clinical appearance of fracture healing in good alignment, full ROM of the knee joints

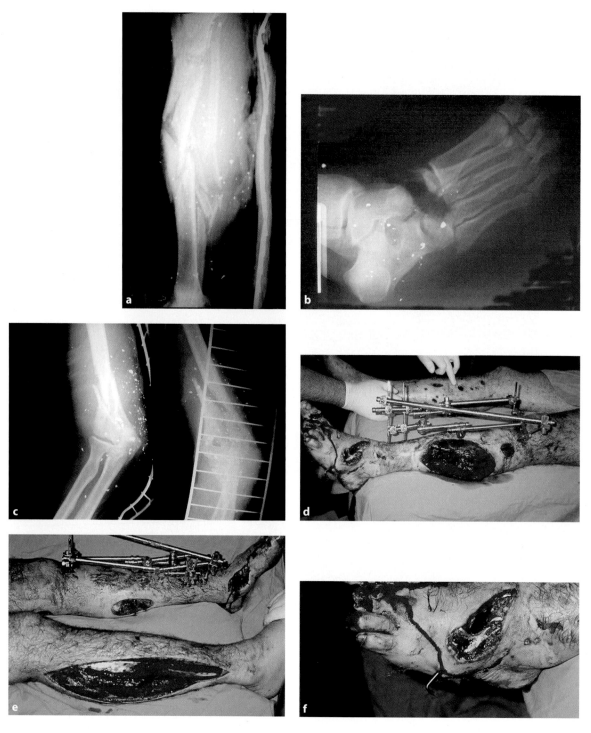

Fig. 3.2.5.4a–z10. A 32-year-old male, victim of a mine explosion, sustained multiple injuries to his left upper limb and bilateral lower limb injuries. After primary medical care on the battlefield he was evacuated by helicopter to our hospital. **a–c** Admission radiographs demonstrated multi-comminuted left tibial fracture; post-traumatic loss of mid-foot bones on left foot; comminuted fracture of left distal humerus and olecranon with radiological signs of many foreign metal bodies in the limb tissues. **d–f** Primary thorough surgical debridement was performed. Right leg fasciotomies were required due to acute compartment syndrome of right leg. Left tibial fracture was stabilized by tubular external fixation frame (Delta configuration), primary fixation of left upper limb fractures with tubular external fixator and temporary elbow bridging. Clinical appearance of the injured limbs after completing primary debridement, fasciotomy of left leg, and primary skeletal stabilization of fractures. Note severe and extensive damage to soft tissues. **g–z10** *see next page*

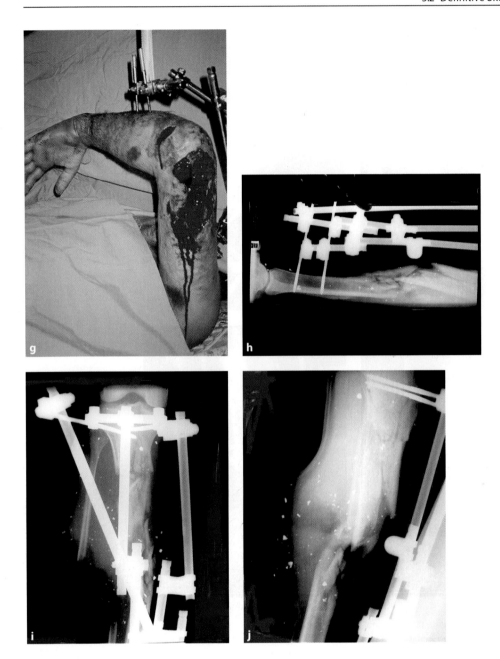

Fig. 3.2.5.4a–z10. *(continued)* **g** Primary thorough surgical debridement was performed. Right leg fasciotomies were required due to acute compartment syndrome of right leg. Left tibial fracture was stabilized by tubular external fixation frame (Delta configuration), primary fixation of left upper limb fractures with tubular external fixator and temporary elbow bridging. Clinical appearance of the injured limbs after completing primary debridement, fasciotomy of left leg, and primary skeletal stabilization of fractures. Note severe and extensive damage to soft tissues. **h–j** Radiographs demonstrated fixation of tibial fracture using tubular frame, bridging of elbow joint; radiological signs of multiple foreign bodies in tissues of the limbs. **k–z10** *see next page*

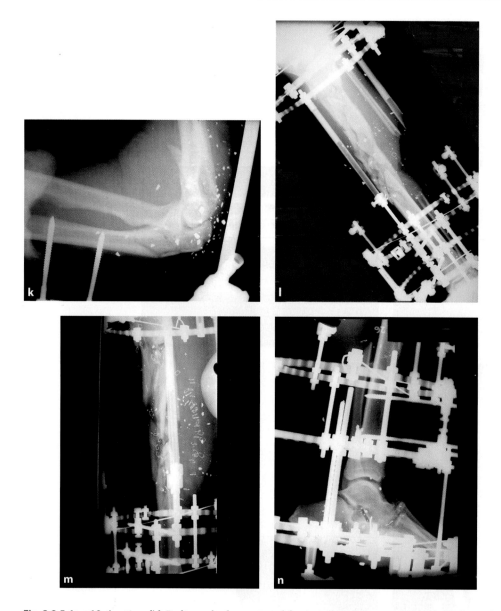

Fig. 3.2.5.4a–z10. *(continued)* **k** Radiographs demonstrated fixation of tibial fracture using tubular frame, bridging of elbow joint; radiological signs of multiple foreign bodies in tissues of the limbs. **l–n** Conversion of tubular external fixators to Ilizarov frames with closed reduction of the fractures using ligamentotaxis and olive wires was performed 6 days later. The left foot with severe bone loss was fixed in a position of acute shortening with bone contact between hind-foot and fore-foot. Postoperative radiological appearance of both legs. Post-traumatic and post-fasciotomy wounds were closed using skin grafts. Clinical appearance of left leg at end of first (**q,r**), second (**s**), and fourth (**t**) weeks after skin grafting. **o–z10** *see next page*

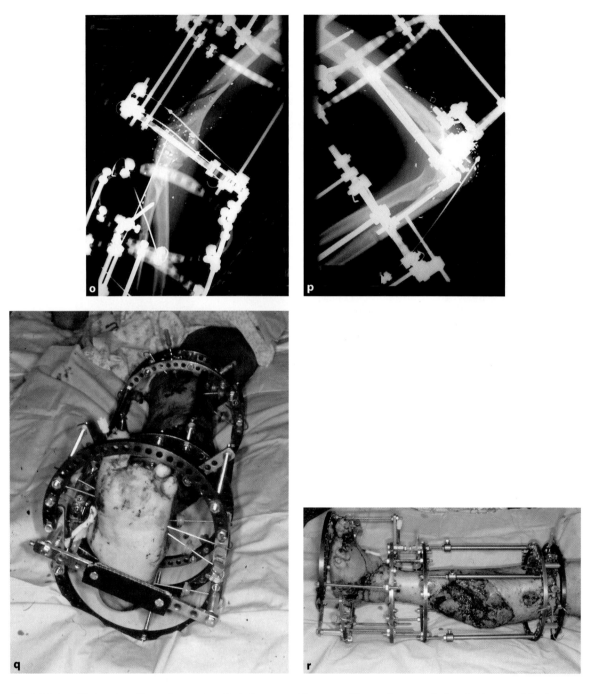

Fig. 3.2.5.4a–z10. *(continued)* **o–p** Conversion of tubular external fixators to Ilizarov frames with closed reduction of the fractures using ligamentotaxis and olive wires was performed 6 days later. The left foot with severe bone loss was fixed in a position of acute shortening with bone contact between hind-foot and fore-foot. Postoperative radiological appearance of both legs. Post-traumatic and post-fasciotomy wounds were closed using skin grafts. Clinical appearance of left leg at end of first (**q,r**), second (**s**), and fourth (**t**) weeks after skin grafting. **s–z10** *see next page*

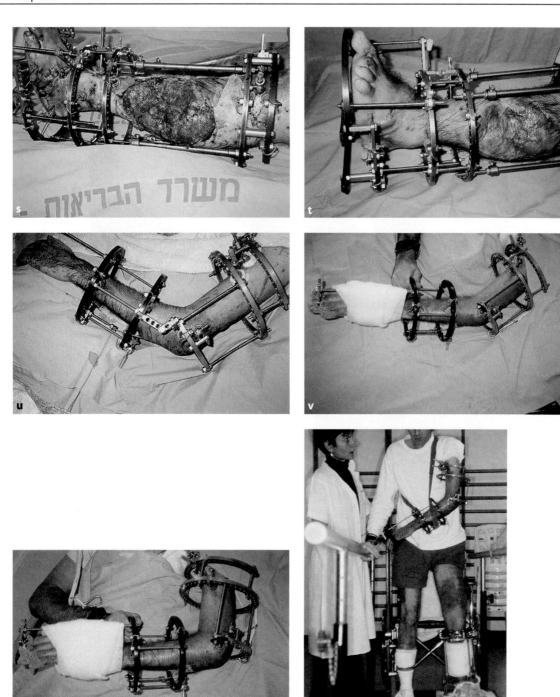

Fig. 3.2.5.4a–z10. *(continued)* Clinical appearance of left leg at end of first (**q,r**), second (**s**), and fourth (**t**) weeks after skin grafting. **u–w** Stabilization of left upper limb factures was performed using hinged Ilizarov external fixation frame with early passive and active mobilization. One month later the hinges were removed. Clinical appearance of the upper limb external fixation. **x** Early standing and walking were permitted in the third week after injury using parallel bars. Clinical photos of rehabilitation stage. **z–z10** *see next page*

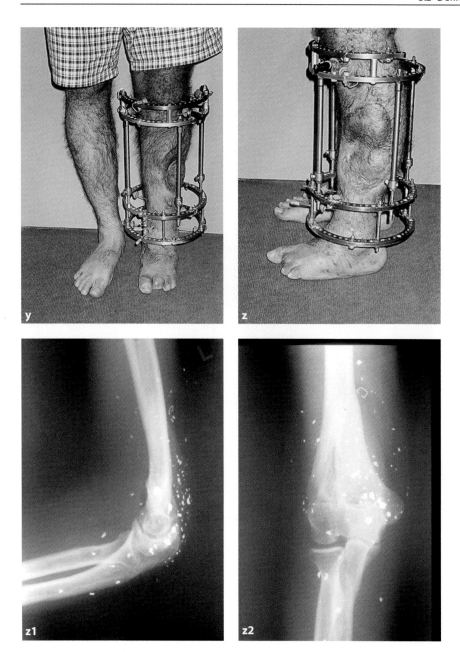

Fig. 3.2.5.4a–z10. *(continued)* **y–z** Early standing and walking were permitted in the third week after injury using parallel bars. Clinical photos of rehabilitation stage. **z1–z2** Time in external fixation of left upper limb and left foot fractures was 4 months. After 10 months of tibial external fixation, radiological signs of solid bone healing were noted, and the Ilizarov frame was removed. Radiological and clinical examination at the 2-year follow-up demonstrates solid bone healing and good functional result. **z3–z10** *see next page*

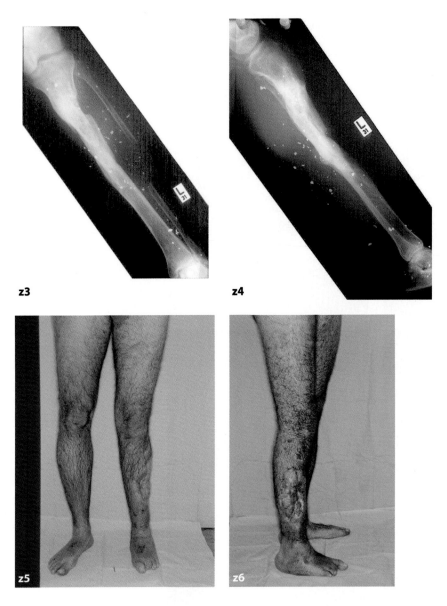

Fig. 3.2.5.4a–z10. *(continued)* **z3–z6** Time in external fixation of left upper limb and left foot fractures was 4 months. After 10 months of tibial external fixation, radiological signs of solid bone healing were noted, and the Ilizarov frame was removed. Radiological and clinical examination at the 2-year follow-up demonstrates solid bone healing and good functional result. **z7–z10** *see next page*

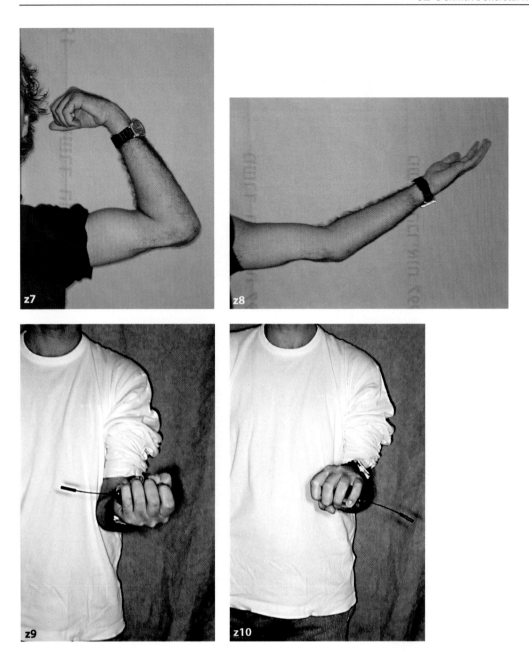

Fig. 3.2.5.4a–z10. (continued) **z7–z10** Time in external fixation of left upper limb and left foot fractures was 4 months. After 10 months of tibial external fixation, radiological signs of solid bone healing were noted, and the Ilizarov frame was removed. Radiological and clinical examination at the 2-year follow-up demonstrates solid bone healing and good functional result. **a,b,h,i,l,n,z3–z6** *Reproduced with permission from © Lippincott Williams and Wilkins; Lerner A et al. (2006) Is staged external fixation a valuable strategy for war injuries to the limbs? Clin Orthop Relat Res 448:217–224 [84].* **c,k,o,u,z7,z8** *Reproduced with permission from © Lippincott Williams and Wilkins; Lerner A et al. (2000) Hybrid external fixation in high energy elbow fractures. A modular system with a promising future. J Trauma 49:1017–1022 [74]*

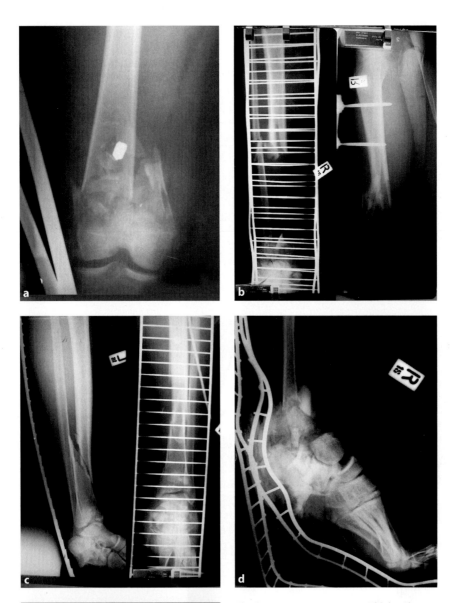

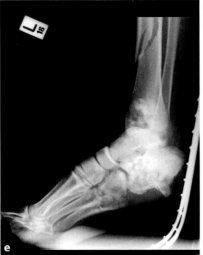

Fig. 3.2.5.5a–z13. A 19-year-old female, victim of a mine explosion due to bus blast, sustained multiple injuries to both lower limbs, including open comminuted supracondylar fracture of right femur, open fracture of right tibia-fibula with traumatic loss of distal half of the tibial bone, open fracture-dislocation of right foot bones with partial loss of calcaneal bone, open pylon fracture of left leg and open fracture of left calcaneus with bone loss. Primary debridement, wound care, and primary external skeletal stabilization using AO tubular frames were performed. Left leg fasciotomies were needed due to acute compartment syndrome of left leg. **a** Admission radiograph demonstrated comminuted supracondylar right femoral fracture with radiological signs of foreign metal body. **b** Radiological appearance of right leg on admission: note loss of the distal half of the tibial bone. **c** Radiological appearance of left leg on admission: note distal tibial fracture with anterior epiphyseal comminuting and bone loss. **d, e** Radiological appearance of both feet on admission: multiple right hind foot fracture-dislocations with partial calcaneal bone loss; left calcaneal fracture with partial bone loss. **f–z13** *see next page*

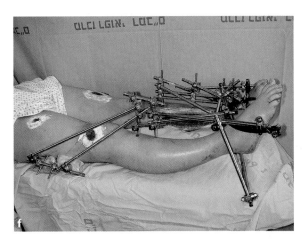

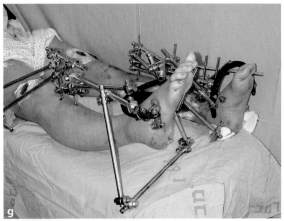

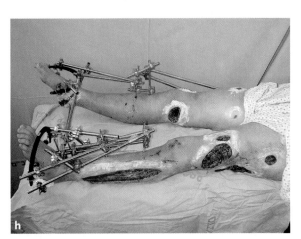

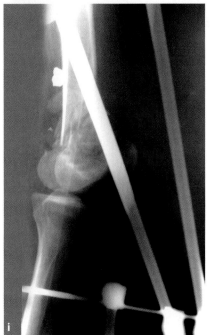

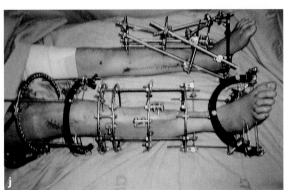

Fig. 3.2.5.5a–z13. *(continued)* **f–h** Primary emergency care was carried out: debridement of soft tissues, left leg fasciotomies, fracture stabilization, including temporary right knee bridging using tubular external fixators with additional hybrid fixation of both feet. Clinical appearance of both lower limbs after completing primary surgical intervention. Note extensive skin and soft-tissue loss over both lower limbs. **i** Radiological appearance of temporary right knee bridging. **j** Conversion of unilateral tubular external fixation on right lower limb to Ilizarov frame and closure of post-fasciotomy wounds of left leg were performed 6 days later. Post-operative clinical appearance of both legs. **k–z13** *see next page*

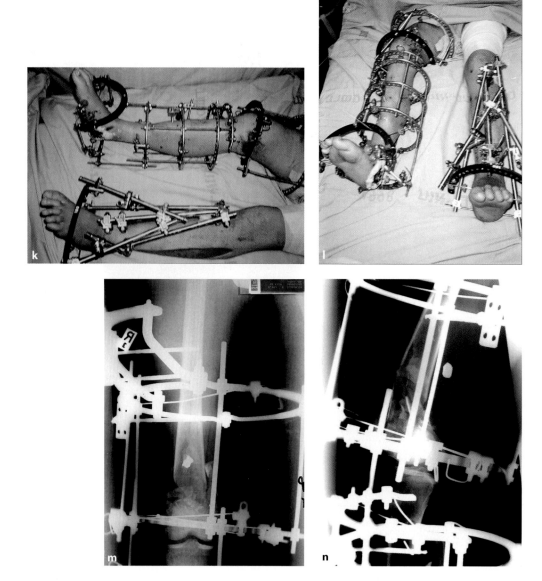

Fig. 3.2.5.5a–z13. *(continued)* **k–l** Conversion of unilateral tubular external fixation on right lower limb to Ilizarov frame and closure of post-fasciotomy wounds of left leg were performed 6 days later. Post-operative clinical appearance of both legs. **m–n** Radiological appearance of right femur and right foot after conversion to Ilizarov fixation. Note that closed reduction of the right foot fracture-dislocation in the Ilizarov frame is successful. **o–z13** *see next page*

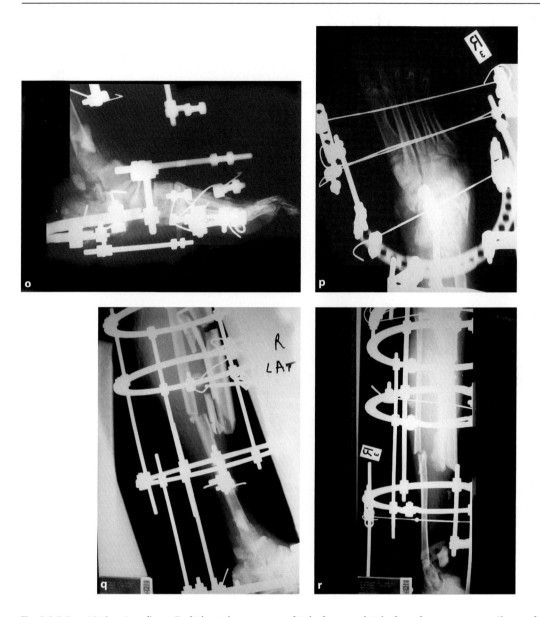

Fig. 3.2.5.5a–z13. *(continued)* **o–p** Radiological appearance of right femur and right foot after conversion to Ilizarov fixation. Note that closed reduction of the right foot fracture-dislocation in the Ilizarov frame is successful. **q,r** On the right leg, after bridging the bone defect in the Ilizarov frame, proximal corticotomy for bone transport is performed. **s–z13** *see next page*

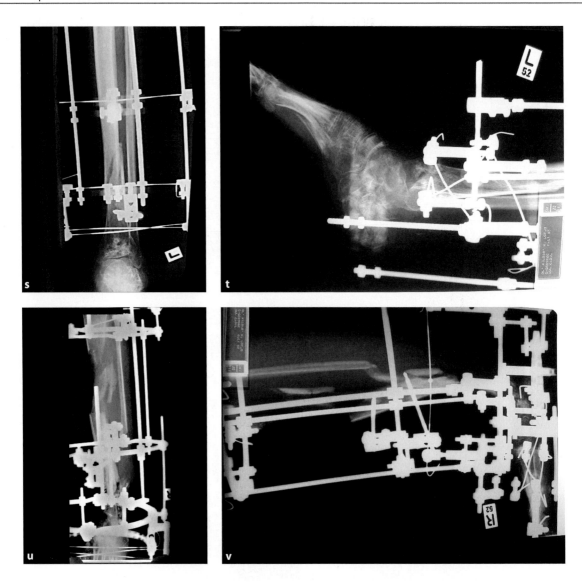

Fig. 3.2.5.5a–z13. *(continued)* **s,t** Radiological appearance of the left leg and foot 3 weeks later. Conversion of unilateral tubular external fixation on the left lower limb to Ilizarov frame is performed at this stage. **u,v** Radiograph after 3 months of bone transport demonstrates weak bone regeneration of the right tibia. **w–z13** *see next page*

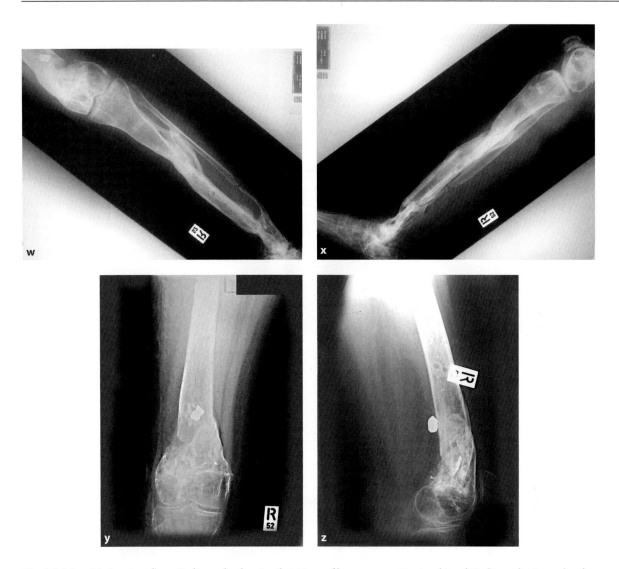

Fig. 3.2.5.5a–z13. *(continued)* **w,x** Radiographs showing that 12 cm of bone regeneration is achieved. Radiograph 12 months after removing the Ilizarov frame demonstrates bone healing in good alignment, with solid bone regeneration at site of bone corticotomy and also tibio-calcaneal fibrous union. Total time in external tibial fixation was 15 months. Patient was fully ambulatory during most of the treatment time. **y,z,** Radiographs 12 months after removing the Ilizarov frame demonstrate bone healing of the right distal femoral fracture, right foot fractures, and left tibial and calcaneal fractures. **z1–z13** *see next page*

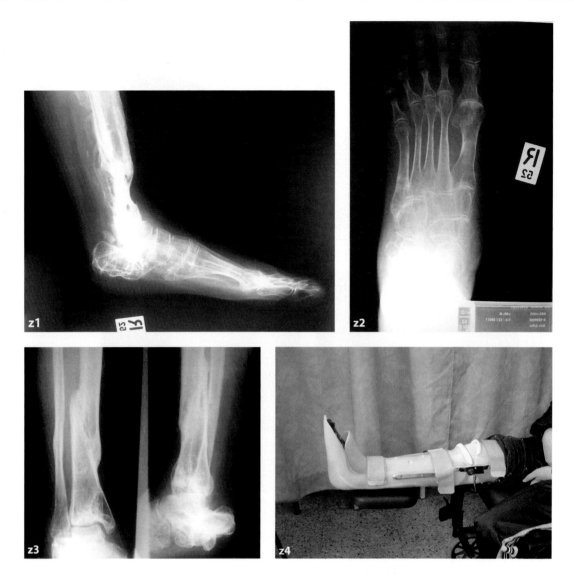

Fig. 3.2.5.5a–z13. *(continued)* **z1–z3** Radiographs 12 months after removing the Ilizarov frame demonstrate bone healing of the right distal femoral fracture, right foot fractures, and left tibial and calcaneal fractures. **z4** During first 6 months after removing the Ilizarov frame, the right lower limb was fixed using a long orthosis with knee hinges (clinical appearance). **z5–z13** *see next page*

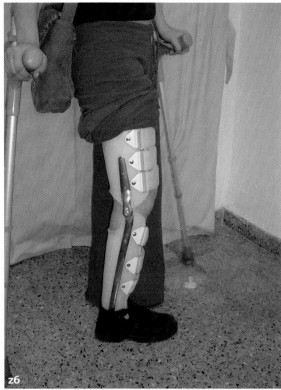

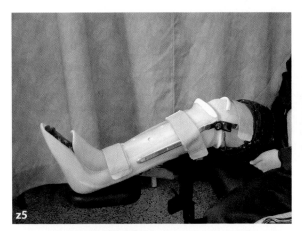

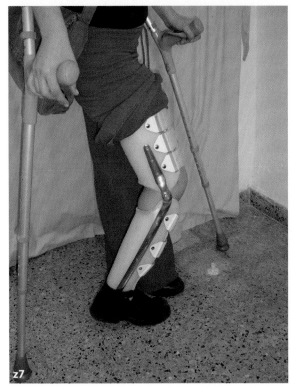

Fig. 3.2.5.5a–z13. *(continued)* **z5** During first 6 months after removing the Ilizarov frame, the right lower limb was fixed using a long orthosis with knee hinges (clinical appearance). **z6**, **z7** Clinical view of the next stage of rehabilitation – walking using functional brace with orthopedic shoe. **z8–z13** *see next page*

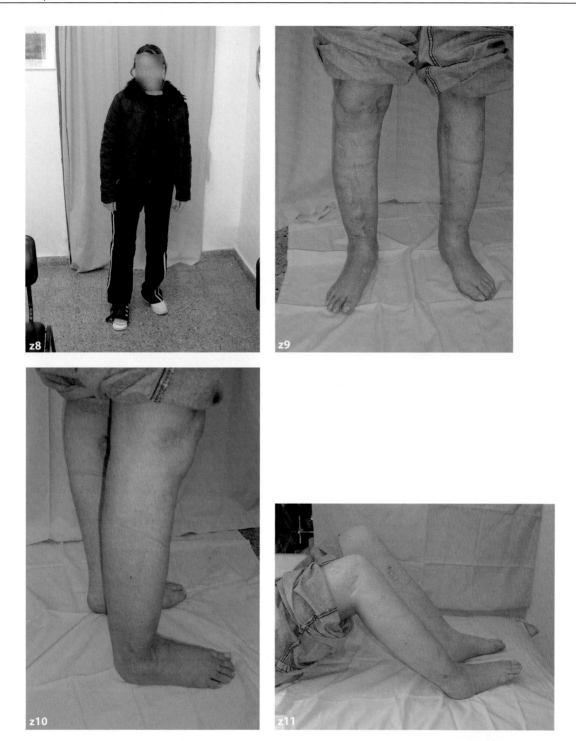

Fig. 3.2.5.5a–z13. *(continued)* **z8–z11** Two-year follow-up: clinical appearance of both legs and standing without additional support. **z12–z13** *see next page*

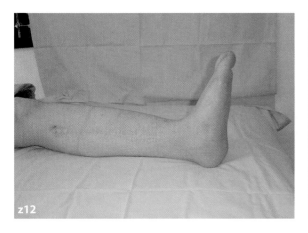
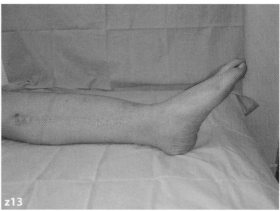

Fig. 3.2.5.5a–z13. *(continued)* **z12–z13** Two-year follow-up: clinical appearance of both legs and standing without additional support

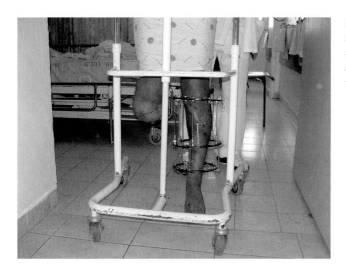

Fig. 3.2.6.1. Clinical appearance of early weight-bearing on single remaining left lower limb. One month after road traffic accident with right below-knee amputation and open Gustilo–Anderson type IIIA left tibial fracture

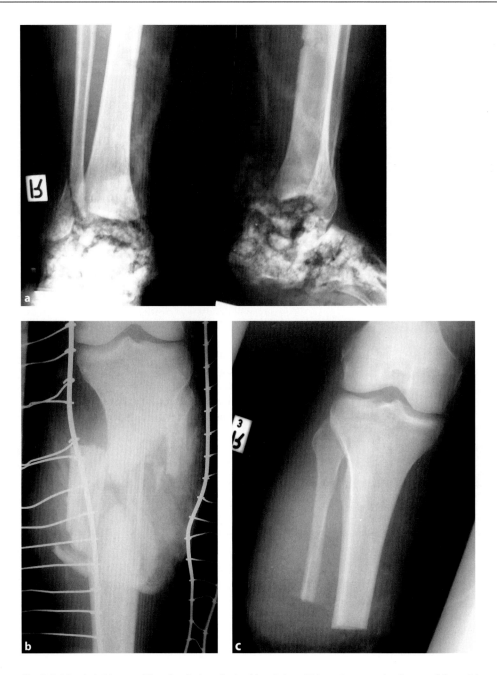

Fig. 3.2.6.2a–j. A 24-year-old male, victim of mine blast injury. This patient sustained severe bilateral lower limb injury with left open fracture of the tibia Gustilo–Anderson type IIIB, and complete destruction of the right foot. **a,b** Radiological appearance of lower limbs on admission. Note severe comminuting and bone loss of left proximal tibia and extreme destruction of right foot and ankle ("bone bag" appearance). **c** Primary debridement of wounds, followed by primary right below-knee amputation. On left leg, immediate skeletal stabilization was performed using unilateral external fixation frame – Delta configuration. Radiological appearance after performing right amputation and external fixation of left tibial fracture. **d–j** *see next page*

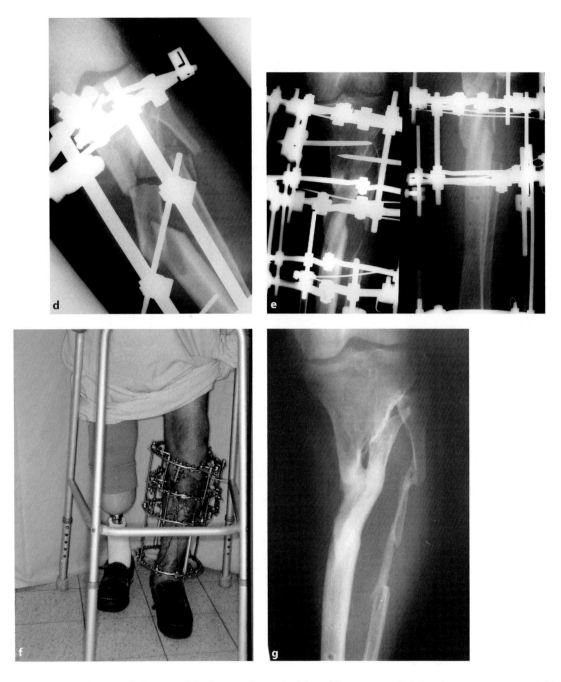

Fig. 3.2.6.2a–j. *(continued)* **d** Primary debridement of wounds, followed by primary right below-knee amputation. On left leg, immediate skeletal stabilization was performed using unilateral external fixation frame – Delta configuration. Radiological appearance after performing right amputation and external fixation of left tibial fracture. **e,f** On 5th day following injury, medial gastrocnemius flap with skin graft to cover extensive anterior soft-tissue defect with exposed bone was performed. The tubular external fixation on the left leg was converted to Ilizarov circular frame. Ten days after conversion to the Ilizarov frame, while commencing the rehabilitation program with full weight-bearing on left leg, the patient was fitted with a prosthesis for the right stump, allowing him to return to erect posture and walking (clinical appearance). Three months later, control radiographs show Ilizarov external fixation of left tibia, with radiological evidence of bone consolidation process and accepted alignment of bone fragments. **g** The Ilizarov frame was removed after 8 months of fixation. On follow-up examination 2 years following injury, the patient was walking freely without aids. Radiological and clinical photos at follow-up demonstrate bone union in acceptable alignment. **h–j** *see next page*

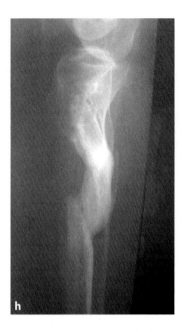
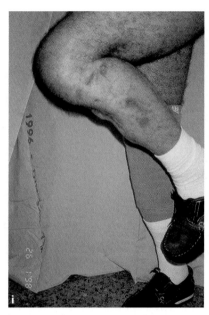
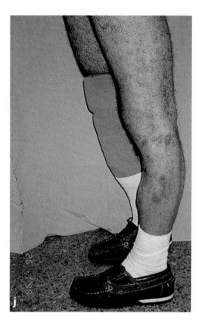

Fig. 3.2.6.2a–j. *(continued)* **h–j** The Ilizarov frame was removed after 8 months of fixation. On follow-up examination 2 years following injury, the patient was walking freely without aids. Radiological and clinical photos at follow-up demonstrate bone union in acceptable alignment. *Reproduced with permission from © Lippincott Williams and Wilkins; Lerner et al. (1998) Ilizarov external fixation in the management of bilateral, highly complex blast injuries of lower extremities: a report of two cases. J Orthop Trauma 12:442–445 [73]*

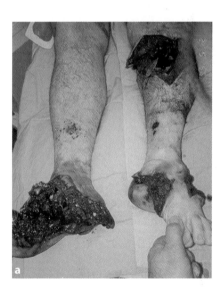
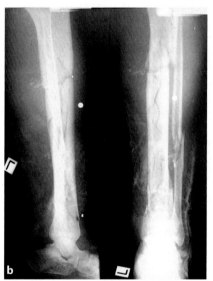

Fig. 3.2.6.3a–c. A 21-year-old male, victim of a mine blast injury. This patient sustained severe bilateral lower limb injury with open fracture of left tibia Gustilo–Anderson type IIIC, and complete destruction of right foot. **a** Clinical appearance of both legs on admission. Note severe extensive damage to soft tissues. **b** Radiological appearance of left leg on admission. Note severe comminuting of left tibia. **c** *see next page*

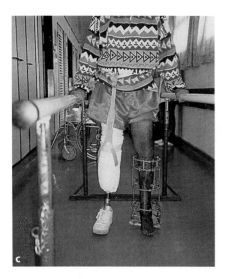

Fig. 3.2.6.3a–c. *(continued)* **c** Patient had primary debridement of wounds, and primary right below-knee amputation was performed. On left leg, primary skeletal stabilization was achieved using unilateral external fixation frame. Immediate vascular repair was performed. After conversion of the unilateral tubular fixation to the Ilizarov frame, the patient began rehabilitation with full weight-bearing on left leg; right leg was fitted with a prosthesis. Clinical appearance of patient walking in parallel bars. Note trans-ankle Ilizarov external stabilization

of arthrodesis has been described, bringing about an evolutionary process of different devices. Large joints are not always easily fused and the most reported techniques possess a significant complications rate, including non-union, infection, and malunion. In complex cases necessitating arthrodesis in the face of severe and extensive bone loss, inadequate soft-tissue coverage, contamination and the presence of foreign bodies (war injuries), the use of internal fixation devices is precluded. The surgical approach here depends on the particular underlying pathologies. Residual cartilage must be excised and meticulous surgical debridement of all non-vital tissues must be performed. The Ilizarov external fixation frame allows sufficient bone and wound stabilization while simultaneously performing arthrodesis of the destroyed joint. The hybrid/circular external fixation is assembled and customized in order to achieve the desired alignment and compression across the fusion site (Fig. 3.2.7.1).

When properly applied, Ilizarov/hybrid frames provide stable immobilization of the joint in three planes with stable fixation against shear and torsion stress, while axial loading is allowed without detrimental effect on the fusion site [58]. This versatile apparatus is highly modular and provides three-dimensional control over bone and joint deformities and instabilities. The frame is usually tailored for the particular patient and may be used for shortening, lengthening, compression, distraction, and bone transport. These parameters are determined intra-operatively but may be repeatedly and reversibly refined postoperatively throughout the healing process in order to eliminate any residual deformity.

Furthermore, this configuration of thin wire frames minimizes surgical invasiveness and provides the surgeon with a remote control over the fused joint. Joint resection is performed using standard techniques. Then the fused joint is temporarily stabilized using two crossed transosseous wires (half-pins). We recommend beginning by mounting the external fixation frame through the insertion of a pair of thin wires around the arthrodesis site: one thin wire from each site. The open operative wound allows insertion of the wires at the required distance from the arthrodesis site and in the correct direction, with a minimal expenditure of time and radiation exposure to the patient and surgical team. These wires are fixed to two rings connected together with threaded rods. Then, the wound is partially closed, leaving a small opening for visual and palpation control of the arthrodesis site during assembly of the fixation frame. This technique has some advantages over the commonly recommended technique of apparatus assembly following skin closure. The first-inserted pair of the thin wires serves as reference points for insertion of the following wires and half-pins during final mounting of the frame. Placement of the proximal and distal rings (or half-rings) of the frame at a distance from the arthrodesis site increases the level of stability of fixation required by the consolidation process. The final closure of the wound and arthrodesis site is performed by placing the last two to three sutures in the skin, whereupon additional thin wires and half-pins are inserted from each ring to further stabilize the fixation frame. The operative procedure is concluded by removing the temporarily placed transfixing wires. Thereafter the compression of the zone of articular resection is performed. All wires and half-pins are inserted extra-focally and, therefore, further damage to the involved tissue is avoided.

In patients with severe shortening due to trauma or as a result of joint fusion, limb length restoration by distraction osteogenesis can be performed at the site

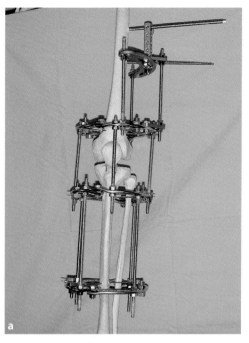
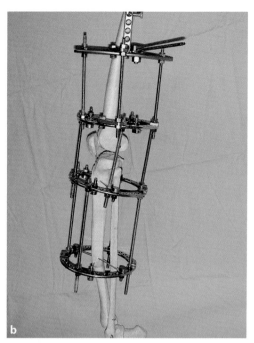
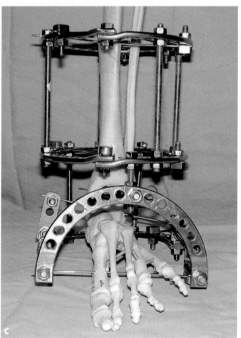
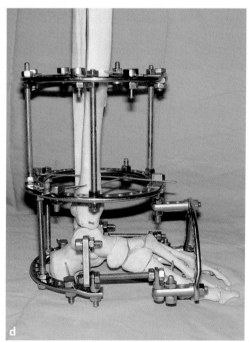

Fig. 3.2.7.1a–d. Ilizarov frame assembly for skeletal stabilization performing fusion procedure. **a,b** Ilizarov fixation frame for knee arthrodesis. **c,d** Ilizarov fixation frame for ankle arthrodesis. *Reproduced with permission from © Acta Orthopaedica Belgica; Calif et al (2004) The Ilizarov external fixation frame in compression arthrodesis of large, weight bearing joints. Acta Orthopaed Belg 70 (1):51–56 [17]*

of fusion or by additional elongation corticotomy/osteotomy. If the shortening is due to post-traumatic and/or post-debridement severe bone loss, it can be repaired using the distraction technique. The method of limb length restoration by distraction osteogenesis at the site of the arthrodesis after 20–30 days of compression is recommended in some publications. We do not recommend this technique in cases of war and other types of severe high-energy injuries because of the low potential for distraction osteogenesis in the tissues in the injury zone. The subsequent bone elongation can be achieved more easily and safely away from the injury site.

Micromovements in the axial plane stimulate bone formation and enhance osseous healing [64]. Hence, early ambulation and weight-bearing are encouraged and may be initiated almost immediately. A permanent compression in the arthrodesis zone must be maintained during the entire period of fixation in the external frame.

After frame removal, all limbs are protected in a plaster of Paris (POP) walking cast for an additional 30 days. (Fig. 3.2.7.2, Fig. 3.2.7.3, Fig. 3.2.7.4)

In patients suffering from high-energy injuries to the elbow joint, with extensive bone and soft-tissue loss, complicated by local infection, all options of surgical reconstruction are precluded, including total elbow arthroplasty. Elbow arthrodesis serves as a salvage option. The modular external fixation frame can be tailored to provide adequate skeletal stabilization in a preferred elbow position for fusion. Gradual sequential adjustment of the frame into 90° flexion can be used in treating patients with severe soft-tissue loss for diminution of a soft-tissue defect and avoiding the need for additional complex skin flap procedures [83] (Fig. 3.2.7.5, Fig. 3.2.7.6).

3.2.8 Primary Circular/Hybrid Fixation Frame Assembly in Emergency Conditions

In the treatment of some patients with severe trauma, contrary to the general principles of our staged protocol, it is possible to avoid the stage of primary temporary simple external fixation and perform the definitive precise reduction and fixation of the bone fragments as the primary surgical procedure. The early reduction of the bone fragments eliminates pressure on the soft tissues and improves conditions for successful healing. Moreover, the need for a secondary operative orthopedic procedure is avoided. This can only be done if the general condition of the patient is stable and concomitant life-threatening injuries are absent. The blood supply to the limb must be adequate: vascular repair can be technically impeded in conditions of the circular frame around the injured limb. The absence of significant soft-tissue defects, demanding local or free tissue transfer for the coverage of the wound, is also a condition

since the circular fixation frame constitutes a technical obstacle in performing these complex procedures. The absence of a well-trained expert in the Ilizarov method is an absolute contraindication to the performance of such a technically difficult and complex procedure in an emergency situation (Fig. 3.2.8.1).

Application of the circular Ilizarov device can be performed step-by-step, if needed. With this method, skeletal stabilization in the alignment position only is performed in the first emergency stage of the treatment. The fixed limb is held in the circular frame in an elevated position, preserving skin and soft tissues on the inferior surface of the limb from any, even minimal, pressure. The next stage of the treatment is final precise reduction and stable fixation of the bone fragments, and is performed only after stabilization of the patient's general and local condition has been achieved (Fig. 3.2.8.2).

Primary reduction and stabilization of bone fragments using a circular or hybrid external fixation frame is indicated for immediate fixation in treating patients suffering from complex severe fractures combined with extensive damage or loss of skin and soft tissues on the posterior surface of the injured limb. The modularity of the hybrid fixators allows the construction of an appropriate frame, combining sufficient bone stabilization and preservation of soft tissues from pressure, and allowing an approach for plastic reconstructive procedures (Fig. 3.2.8.3).

3.3 Limb Salvage in Severe Bone and Soft-Tissue Loss

3.3.1 Bone Reconstruction by Callotasis

High-energy limb trauma may be accompanied by extensive bone loss, demanding complex measures to replace and restore length and configuration to the injured bone. Bone loss may occur from extrusion of bone fragments at the time of injury, during debridement of the open fracture when devitalized segments of the bone are removed, or as a result of both these mechanisms, thereby creating a defect [63, 69]. Severe damage to soft tissues complicates the resolution of the bone loss situation [76, 120, 122]. Especially in the treatment of combat trauma (gunshot wounds and blast injuries), foreign bodies are present in the tissues, which significantly increases the hazard of post-traumatic local sepsis. All these factors have a negative effect on the suitability of bone grafting. In contrast, the method of controlled gradual distraction of bone fragments stabilized and fixed in the external fixation frame utilizes the osteogenic properties of the existing bone, not only for the fracture healing process, but also for filling of the bone defects. Soft-tissue tension during distraction in the frame also has some stabilizing effect

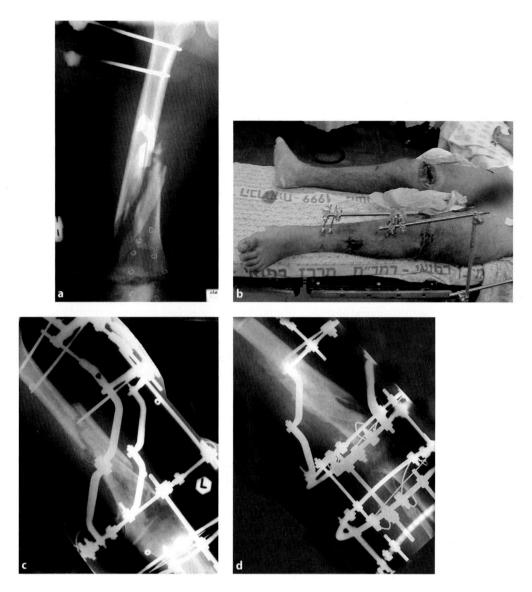

Fig. 3.2.7.2a–r. A 30-year-old male, victim of road traffic accident. This patient sustained bilateral lower limb injuries with open fracture of the left femur Gustilo–Anderson type IIIB with primary articular bone loss, left tibial fracture Gustilo–Anderson type IIIA, and closed right tibial plateau fracture. The patient had primary debridement of wounds, followed by skeletal stabilization using a unilateral external fixation frame with knee joint bridging. **a** Radiological appearance of left femoral fracture with tubular trans-knee external fixation. Note knee articular bone destruction. **b** Clinical appearance of both injured legs after debridement of wounds and performing of left trans-knee external fixation. **c–d** One week later, repeated debridement of wounds with conversion of the tubular fixation to Ilizarov circular frames. Postoperative radiograph showing an Ilizarov external fixation of left femur and left tibia, trans-knee rigid fixation after resection of the knee articular surface. **e–r** *see next page*

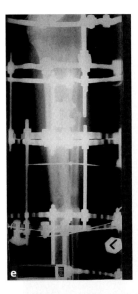

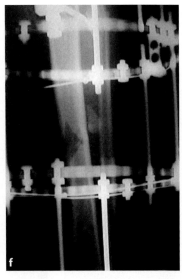

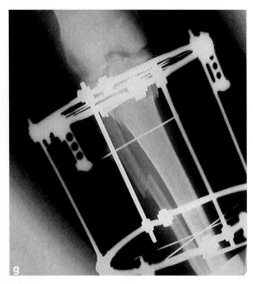

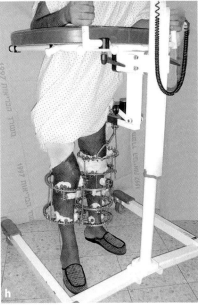

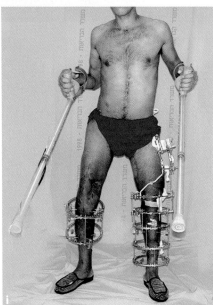

Fig. 3.2.7.2a–r. *(continued)* **e–f** One week later, repeated debridement of wounds with conversion of the tubular fixation to Ilizarov circular frames. Postoperative radiograph showing an Ilizarov external fixation of left femur and left tibia, trans-knee rigid fixation after resection of the knee articular surface. **g** Radiological appearance of the right tibial bone after performing closed reduction and minimal internal fixation using two cannulated screws, and additional external support using Ilizarov frame. **h–i** Clinical photos demonstrate full weight-bearing using walker and crutches from the first days after surgery. **j–r** *see next page*

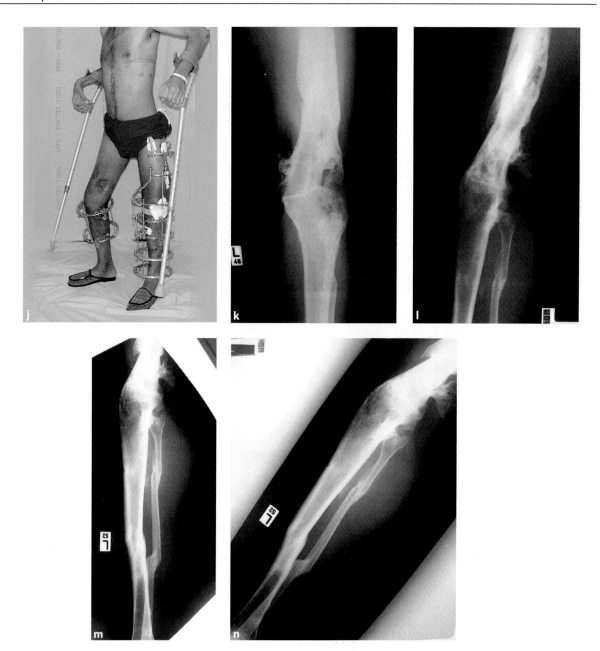

Fig. 3.2.7.2a–r. *(continued)* **j** Clinical photos demonstrate full weight-bearing using walker and crutches from the first days after surgery. **k–n** Ilizarov external fixation frame was removed after 4 months from the right tibia, and after 6 months from the left lower limb. Follow-up at 18 months: fractures of both legs are healed and knee arthrodesis is achieved. **o–r** *see next page*

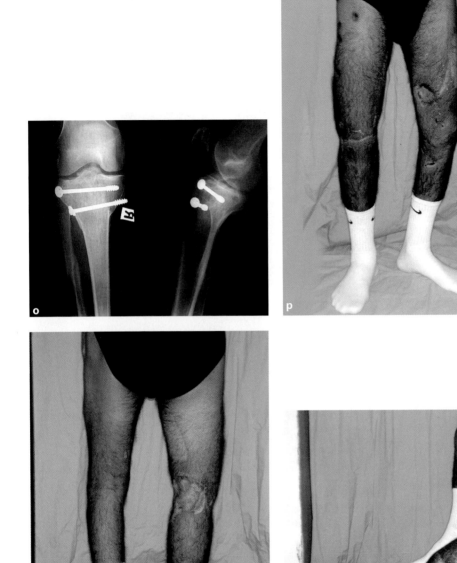

Fig. 3.2.7.2a–r. *(continued)* **o** Ilizarov external fixation frame was removed after 4 months from the right tibia, and after 6 months from the left lower limb. Follow-up at 18 months: fractures of both legs are healed and knee arthrodesis is achieved. **p–r** Clinical appearance at follow-up at 18 months

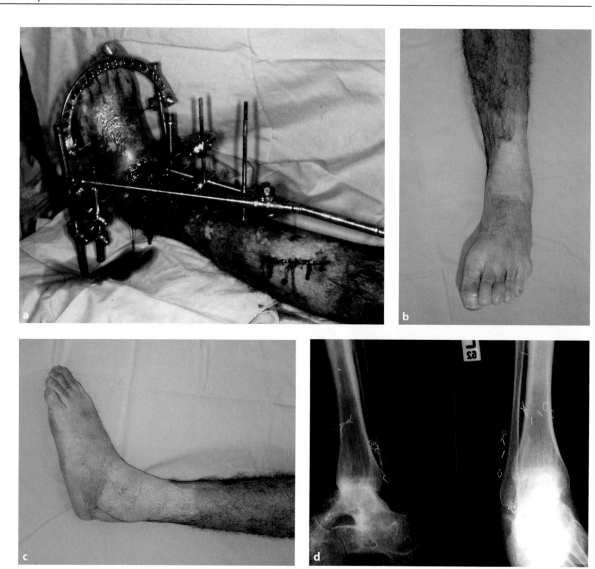

Fig. 3.2.7.3a–d. A 19-year-old victim of motorcycle road accident with open fracture dislocation of the left ankle with soft-tissue defect above the anterior aspect of ankle joint and extensive chondral loss of the distal tibia and talus. Radical debridement and immediate trans-ankle stabilization using a hybrid external fixation frame were performed (primary arthrodesis). **a** Clinical photo demonstrates anterior view after completing primary debridement and stabilization. **b,c** Coverage of the exposed ankle was performed 5 days later, using free latissimus dorsi muscle flap. Clinical photo at follow-up 2 years later demonstrates good skin and soft-tissue appearance. **d** Radiological appearance at follow-up 2 years later demonstrates solid tibio-talo-calcaneal fusion

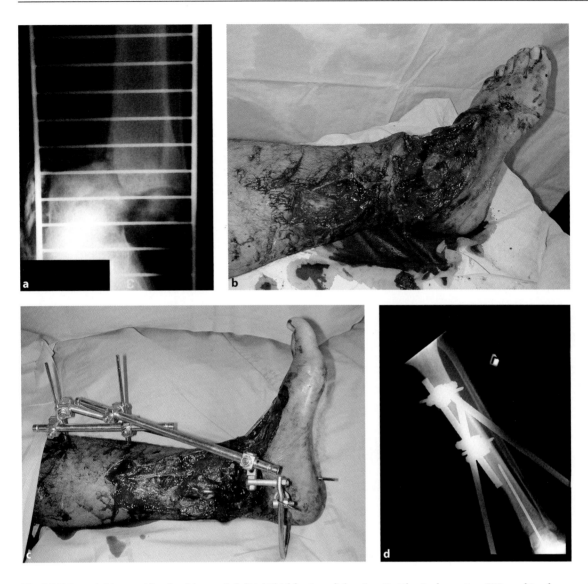

Fig. 3.2.7.4a–s. A 24-year-old male with open left distal tibial fracture-dislocation Gustilo–Anderson type IIIB resulting from crush injury due to work accident. **a** Admission radiographs. Radiological signs of fracture-dislocation of the ankle joint. **b** Clinical appearance of left leg on admission. Note extensive skin and soft-tissue loss over distal third of the leg and ankle joint. **c** Patient had primary debridement of wounds. Skeletal stabilization was performed using hybrid external fixation frame. Clinical appearance of the leg after completing primary operative procedure. **d** Control postoperative radiograph of the leg. **e–s** *see next page*

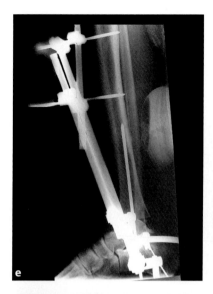
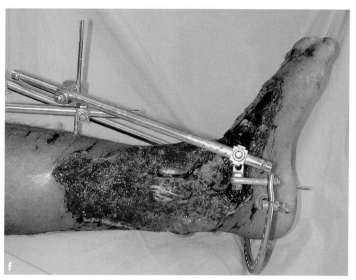
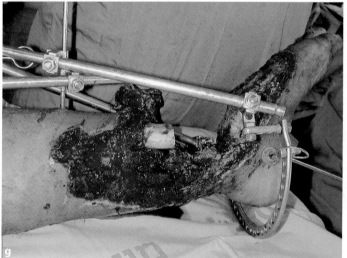
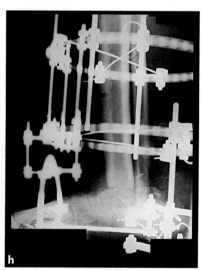

Fig. 3.2.7.4a–s. *(continued)* **e** Control postoperative radiograph of the leg. **f** Clinical appearance on 5th day after trauma. Note severe post-traumatic necrosis in the zone of injury. **g** Clinical appearance of the leg after performing radical necrectomy with resection of the necrotic bone end of the tibial bone and astragalectomy (total 13 cm). **h** Acute shortening performed to diminish soft-tissue defect after radical necrectomy. Radiological appearance of bone contact between resected tibial bone and calcaneus. **i–s** *see next page*

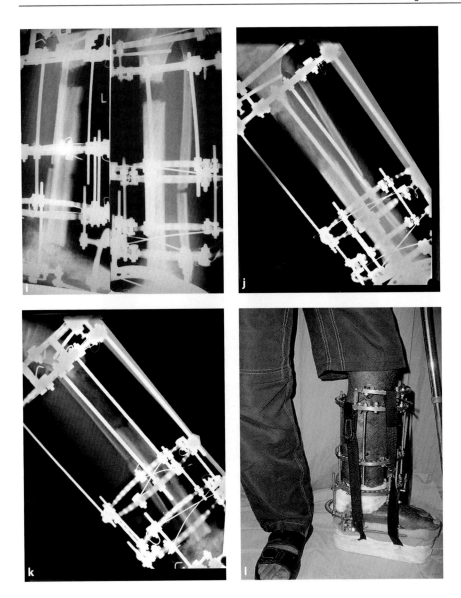

Fig. 3.2.7.4a–s. *(continued)* **i** Three weeks later, after healing of soft-tissue wound, proximal tibial corticotomy was performed to eliminate distal tibial bone defect using a bone transport technique. Radiograph taken 1 month after corticotomy demonstrates tibial bone transport. **j,k** Radiological appearance of bone regeneration 3 months after corticotomy. **l** Early full weight-bearing allowed during entire period of stabilization and elongation in the external fixation frame. **m–s** *see next page*

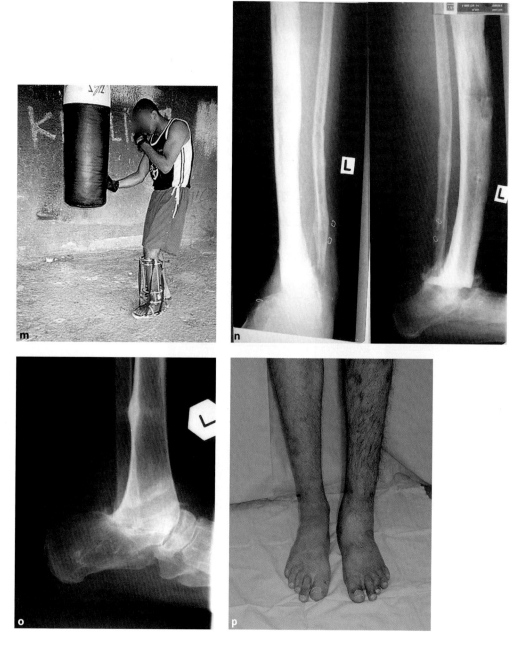

Fig. 3.2.7.4a–s. *(continued)* **m** Early full weight-bearing allowed during entire period of stabilization and elongation in the external fixation frame. **n** Ilizarov frame was removed after 15 months of external fixation. After removing the Ilizarov frame, functional loading was continued using walking brace. Note radiological appearance of solid bone regeneration. **o** Radiological appearance of solid bone tibio-calcaneal fusion. **p** Clinical appearance on follow-up 2 years after removing the Ilizarov fixation frame. **q–s** *see next page*

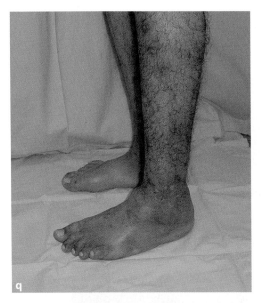

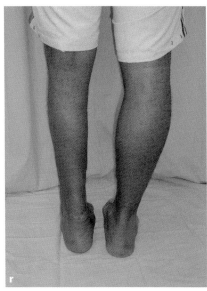

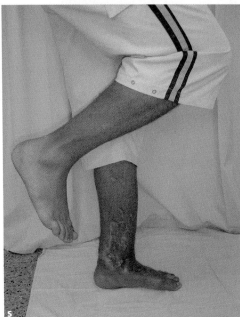

Fig. 3.2.7.4a–s. *(continued)* **q–s** Clinical appearance on follow-up 2 years after removing the Ilizarov fixation frame

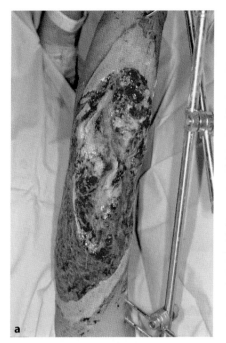

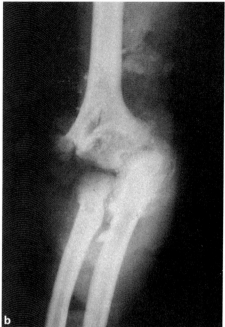

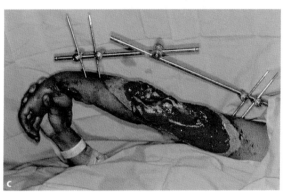

Fig. 3.2.7.5a–h. An 18-year-old male driver involved in a side-impact collision with a tree, sustaining a severe high-energy "sideswipe" injury. The extensive bone and soft-tissue loss and local infection precluded restoration of the articular anatomy. **a** Clinical appearance of the posterior aspect of the elbow joint. Note extensive soft-tissue loss with exposed elbow joint. **b** Radiograph of destroyed elbow joint on admission. Note severe bone damage to distal humeral, proximal ulnar, and radial bones. **c** Primary emergency care was carried out, with debridement of soft tissues and stabilization of the elbow by temporary bridging. Clinical appearance of the tubular external fixation frame provided primary skeletal stabilization. **d–h** *see next page*

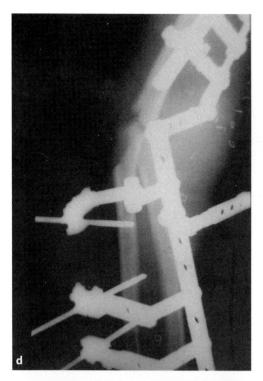

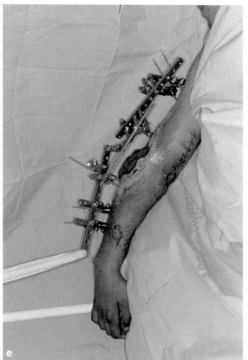

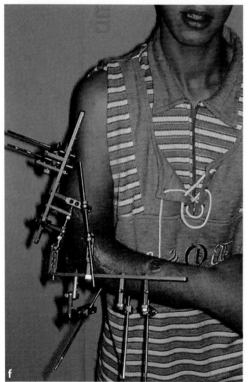

Fig. 3.2.7.5a–h. *(continued)* **d,e** A large area on the posterior aspect of the elbow (approximately 200 cm²) was rendered deficient in soft-tissue coverage. Persistent local infection with drainage precluded tissue transfer. Primary elbow arthrodesis using external fixation frame was the only option. The rigid tubular trans-elbow frame was exchanged at this stage for a unilateral hinged frame. The frame was primarily locked in a position of elbow extension, a maneuver that immediately diminished the posterior soft-tissue defect to approximately 60 cm². Clinical and radiological appearance of the elbow after application of a unilateral hinged external fixation frame that transfixed the elbow joint. **f** The modular frame provides not only skeletal stability and local wound care, but also postoperative stepwise flexion of the elbow toward a functional flexion position, maintaining compression at the arthrodesis site. The residual wound healed uneventfully by secondary intention. Clinical and radiological photos taken 3 weeks following hinged frame application demonstrates the achievement of 80° elbow flexion. **g–h** *see next page*

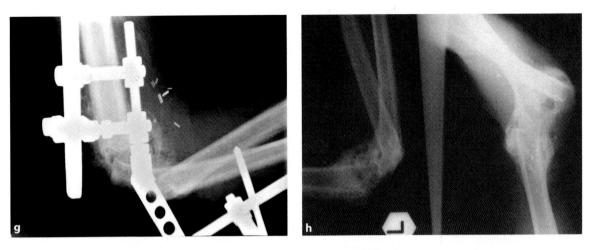

Fig. 3.2.7.5a–h. *(continued)* **g** The modular frame provides not only skeletal stability and local wound care, but also postoperative stepwise flexion of the elbow toward a functional flexion position, maintaining compression at the arthrodesis site. The residual wound healed uneventfully by secondary intention. Clinical and radiological photos taken 3 weeks following hinged frame application demonstrates the achievement of 80° elbow flexion. **h** Radiological pictures showing solid bony fusion attained within 2 months. **b–d, f,h** *Reproduced with permission from © Lippincott Williams and Wilkins; Lerner et al. (2005) Unilateral, hinged external fixation frame for elbow compression arthrodesis: the stepwise attainment of a stable 90-degree flexion position. A case report. J Orthop Trauma 19:52–55 [83]*

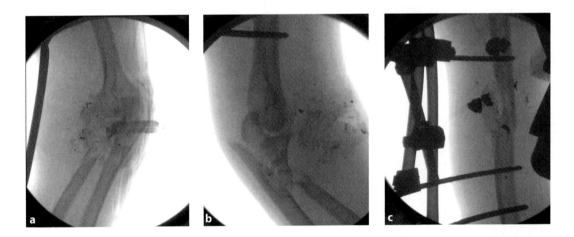

Fig. 3.2.7.6a–n. A 20-year-old male with open Gustilo–Anderson type IIIB fractures of right humeral shaft, right proximal ulnar and radial bones with severe bone comminuting, and bone and soft-tissue loss due to gunshot injury. Primary treatment included debridement of wounds with external fixation of fractures, including elbow bridging using tubular external fixation frame. **a–c** Radiographs of destroyed elbow joint after completing the primary stabilization procedure. Note severe bone comminuting and the presence of multiple foreign bodies. **d–n** *see next page*

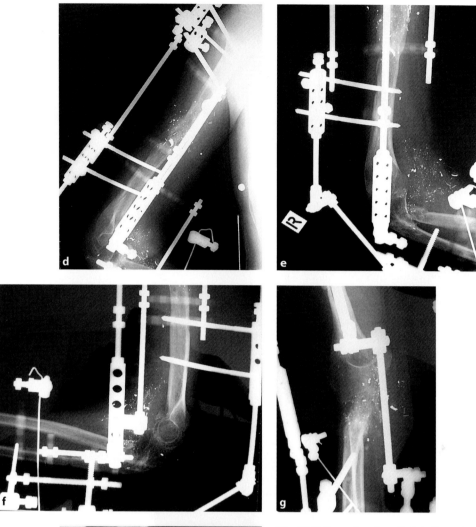

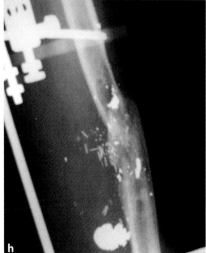

Fig. 3.2.7.6a–n. *(continued)* **d–h** Extensive bone comminuting combined with severe soft-tissue, including neuromuscular, damage. Unstable general condition of the patient precluded an elbow joint reconstructive procedure. Seven days later, the tubular trans-elbow frame was exchanged for a circular fixation frame. Radiological appearance of the elbow after application of a circular external fixation frame for stabilization of fractures and stable fixation of the elbow joint in a 90° position for arthrodesis. **i–n** *see next page*

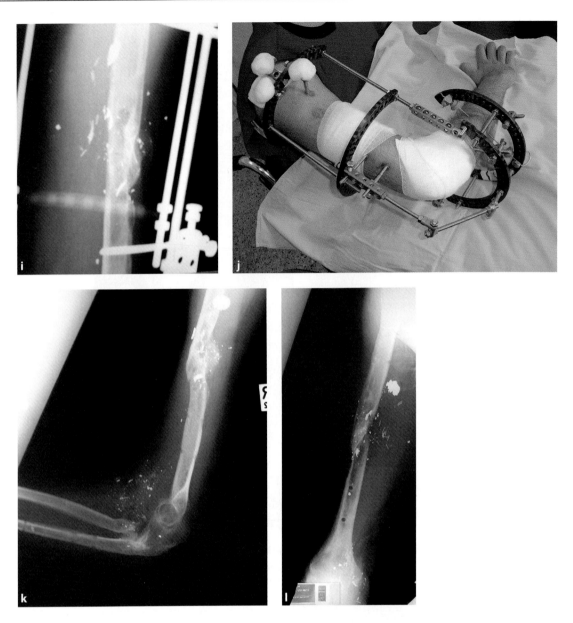

Fig. 3.2.7.6a–n. *(continued)* **i** Extensive bone comminuting combined with severe soft-tissue, including neuromuscular, damage. Unstable general condition of the patient precluded an elbow joint reconstructive procedure. Seven days later, the tubular trans-elbow frame was exchanged for a circular fixation frame. Radiological appearance of the elbow after application of a circular external fixation frame for stabilization of fractures and stable fixation of the elbow joint in a 90° position for arthrodesis. **j** Clinical picture demonstrates Ilizarov external fixation frame in 90° of elbow flexion. **k–l** Radiological appearance after removing Ilizarov frame demonstrates solid consolidation of upper limb fractures and presence of post-traumatic fibrous elbow joint ankylosis. **m–n** *see next page*

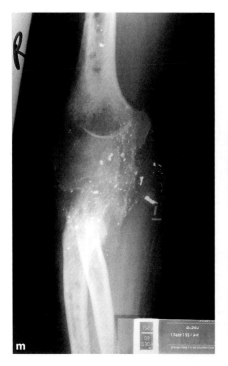

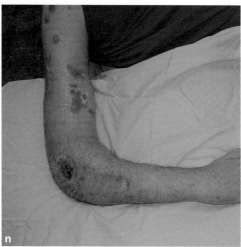

Fig. 3.2.7.6a–n. *(continued)* **m** Radiological appearance after removing Ilizarov frame demonstrates solid consolidation of upper limb fractures and presence of post-traumatic fibrous elbow joint ankylosis. **n** Clinical appearance after removing Ilizarov frame demonstrates post-traumatic fibrous elbow joint fusion in 90° position

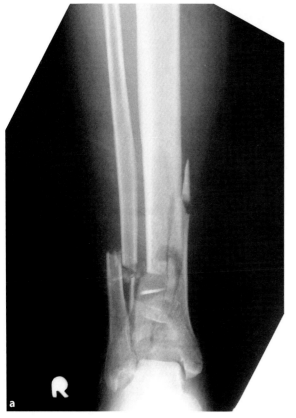

Fig. 3.2.8.1a–p. A 58-year-old male with closed right pylon fracture with severe bone comminuting due to fall from 3 m was referred from another hospital with half-pin inserted for skeletal traction to the calcaneal bone. **a** Radiological appearance on admission to our hospital. Note severe bone comminuting and displacing of distal tibial bone fragments with destruction of articular surface. **b–p** *see next page*

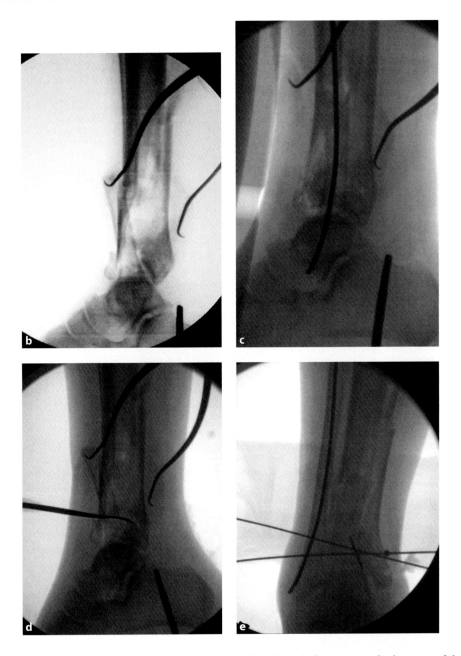

Fig. 3.2.8.1a–p. *(continued)* **b** Intra-operative lateral radiograph demonstrates displacement of the intra-articular anterior bone fragment. **c** After reduction of displaced bone fragments, fibular bone is fixed using intramedullary placed rush pin. **d** Radiograph demonstrates process of reduction of the displaced intra-articular fragments using small surgical periosteal elevator. **e** Articular roof of the ankle joint is fixed using subchondrally placed thin wires, including olive wires. **f–p** *see next page*

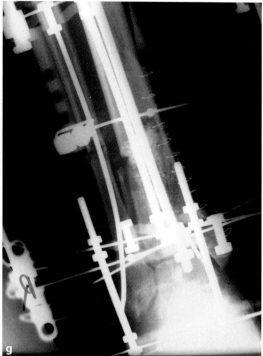

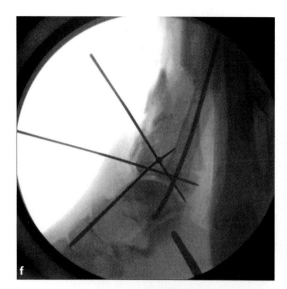

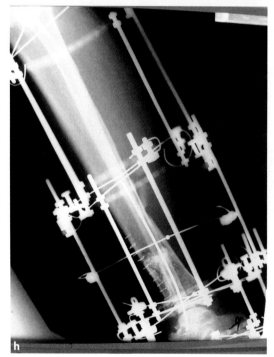

Fig. 3.2.8.1a–p. f Thin wires are used for additional fixation of bone fragments during repositioning procedure. Calcium-phosphate was used for filling of bone loss. **g,h** Postoperative radiographs demonstrate reconstruction of articular surface with good alignment of the tibial shaft. **i–p** *see next page*

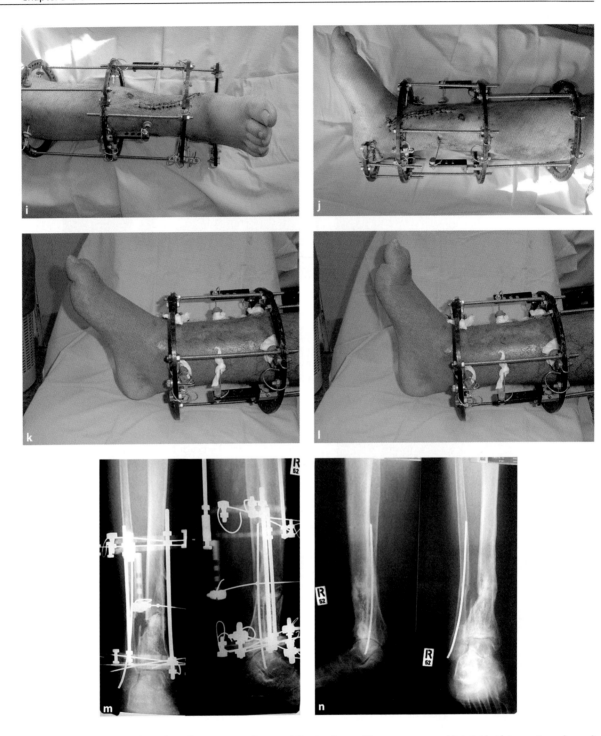

Fig. 3.2.8.1a–p. *(continued)* **i,j** Clinical appearance of external fixation frame. Note temporary ankle joint bridging, using calcaneal half-ring with thin wires. **k,l** Calcaneal half-ring removed after 6 weeks of trans-fixation. Clinical appearance of active motions after removing calcaneal half-ring. **m** Radiological signs of bone healing after 6 months of external fixation. **n** After 1 month more of external fixation, the Ilizarov frame was removed. Radiographs 18 months after removing the Ilizarov frame demonstrate bone healing of the fracture in good alignment with preservation of the articular surface. **o,p** *see next page*

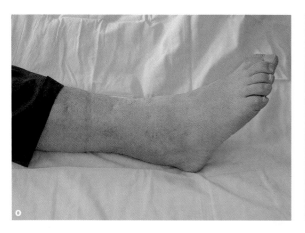
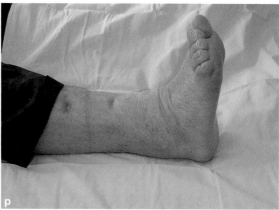

Fig. 3.2.8.1a–p. *(continued)* **o,p** Clinical pictures at follow-up 18 months after removal of the Ilizarov frame

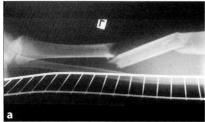
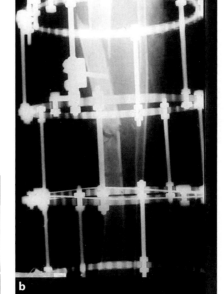

Fig. 3.2.8.2a–i. A 28-year-old male with open left segmental tibial fracture Gustilo–Anderson type IIIA with acute compartment syndrome and closed right tibial fracture due to traffic accident as a pedestrian. Primary debridement and fasciotomy of the left leg were performed immediately. Closed reduction and fixation using unreamed intramedullary nailing were performed on the right leg. **a** Radiograph of displaced segmental tibial fracture of left leg. **b** Re-alignment and primary stabilization of left tibial fracture, using Ilizarov frame with five rings. Anatomical reduction of bone fragments is adjourned until stabilization of local tissue condition. **c–i** *see next page*

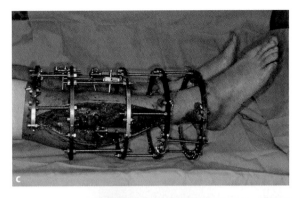

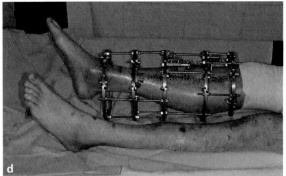

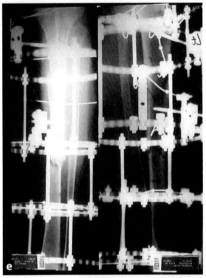

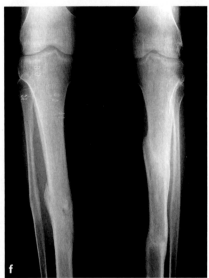

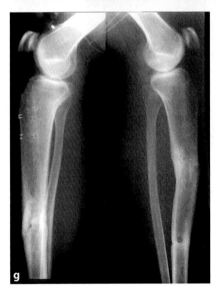

Fig. 3.2.8.2a–i. *(continued)* **c,d** Closure of medial wound using secondary sutures and lateral wound using skin graft is performed. Clinical appearance (medial and lateral aspects). **e** Anatomical reduction and stable fixation of bone fragments is performed in a closed manner using additional pulling olive wires and half-pins. Radiographs demonstrate anatomical reduction of the fracture. **f,g** Six months later, the Ilizarov fixation frame was removed. Removing the intramedullary nail from the right tibia was performed 8 months after the trauma. Radiological appearance of both legs 5 years after the trauma demonstrates solid bone healing in good alignment. **h,i** *see next page*

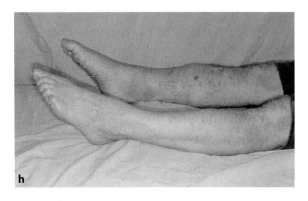
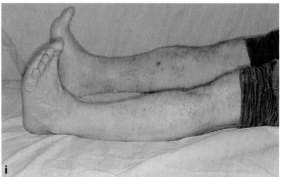

Fig. 3.2.8.2a–i. (continued) **h,i** Clinical appearance at 5-year follow-up

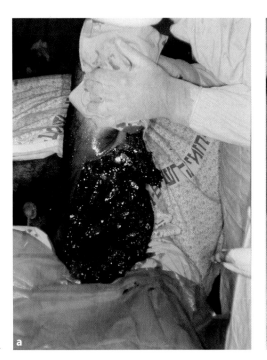
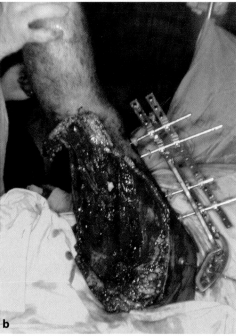

Fig. 3.2.8.3a–c. A 19-year-old male with open fracture of the femoral shaft and extensive soft tissue loss on posterior aspects of the thigh due to blast injury by anti-tank rocket. **a** Clinical appearance of lower limb on admission to hospital. Note extensive destruction of soft tissue on the posterior aspect of the thigh. **b** Clinical view after soft-tissue debridement and unilateral external fixation of the femoral fracture. **c** *see next page*

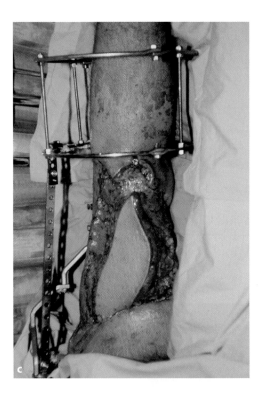

Fig. 3.2.8.3a–c. *(continued)* **c** Clinical appearance after coverage of the wound with free latissimus dorsi muscle flap (central) and skin grafts (peripheral). Unilateral external fixation frame was converted to a circular Ilizarov frame with temporary bridging of knee joint

on the overall fixation system. Callotasis is successfully utilized in elective orthopedics for limb elongation using osteotomy or corticotomy, and also for restoring the length and shape of the bone in the treatment of fractures caused by low-energy trauma in the presence of sufficient blood circulation in the fracture zone. Severe high-energy limb trauma, especially crush injuries and war trauma producing significant destruction of the periosteal soft tissues and damaging the blood supply to the fracture site, causes considerable reduction of the local osteogenic potential and often excludes the possibilities of using it for elongation and bone defect restoration. In the treatment of patients suffering from high-energy limb trauma, we believe that it is possible to employ the method of callotasis only in the presence of well-vascularized coverage of the fracture site, good contact between bone fragments, and with a relatively small extent of bone tissue loss (up to 3-cm-long defects). Metaphyseal localization of the fracture is preferred for this procedure. The very low regenerative potential of the tissues in a zone of high-energy limb trauma can require significantly more time to achieve solid bone consolidation, and, accordingly, prolonged terms of fixation in the external frame. In patients in

whom the radiological appearance of a weak bone regenerate is present, the rate of bone distraction must be decreased or temporarily ceased, and a temporary return to compression of the regenerated bone may be required. This procedure (accordion maneuver) can be performed repeatedly until attainment of the positive effect is shown on the control radiographs.

In conclusion, the procedure of callotasis has a very limited use in the treatment of patients suffering from high-energy limb trauma, due to the decreased reparative potential of the severely injured tissues. It is desirable to perform major reconstruction in relatively healthy tissue zones, moving away from the maximal tissue damage location (Fig. 3.3.1.1).

3.3.2 Bone Reconstruction Using Bifocal Technique

The absence of sufficient vascular coverage of the fracture site, the lack of a good contact between the bone fragments, the considerable loss of bone tissues (more than 2–3 cm), and the diaphyseal localization of the fractures mean that regenerative tissue potential in the fracture zone will be insufficient not only for distractional osteogenesis but also for solid fracture healing. Diaphyseal high-energy fractures of the lower extremities with extensive soft tissue and bone loss, either through the wound or after radical debridement, are the most common indications for using the bifocal method of treatment.

Primary fracture stabilization using a unilateral external frame facilitates soft-tissue care and patient mobilization. The second stage of the treatment (conversion to a circular frame and corticotomy) can be accomplished on an elective basis after thorough preoperative planning. According to Lowenberg et al. [89], the Ilizarov method has provided the most reliable way of restoring bony continuity in a segmental defect and maintaining equal limb lengths. Optimal bone regeneration can be achieved by using osteotomy/corticotomy through a healthy area of bone in a zone of intact soft tissues, desirably metaphyseal in location, preserving the periosteum, and away from the injury zone. The proximal metaphyseal location is usually preferable to the distal metaphysis because of a better bone regeneration potential [57]. The technique of osteotomy/corticotomy is a matter of great importance, because the bone healing process must occur in the osteotomy site. Therefore, it is necessary to give preference to the "low-energy technique" of bone cutting, especially when treating the consequences of high-energy trauma. The minimally invasive corticotomy technique that respects the vascular supply of the bone by endosteal and periosteal vessels is preferable. The bone cutting techniques that cause considerable damage to the bone will delay or even prevent the process of bone regeneration. The

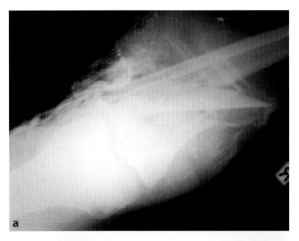
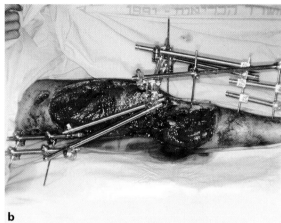
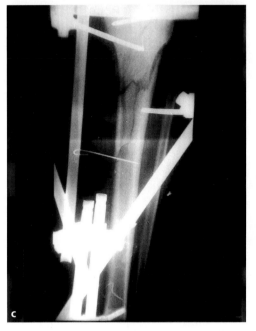
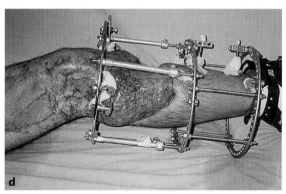

Fig. 3.3.1.1a–t. A 19-year-old male with open Gustilo type IIIB left proximal tibial fracture with severe bone comminuting and massive soft-tissue loss due to blast injury by anti-tank rocket. **a** Radiograph at time of injury. Note severe bone comminuting of the proximal tibial bone. **b,c** Primary emergency care was carried out with debridement of soft tissues and stabilization of the fracture, including temporary knee bridging, using a tubular external fixator. Clinical and radiological appearance of the left lower limb after completing primary surgical intervention. Note extensive skin and soft-tissue loss over the distal third of the left thigh, knee joint, and proximal half of the left leg. **d** Free tissue muscle latissimus dorsi flap and local muscle gastrocnemius flap were used to cover the exposed bone and fracture site. The unilateral tubular trans-knee frame was exchanged at this stage for a circular tibial Ilizarov frame with freeing of the knee joint. Clinical appearance showed complete soft-tissue coverage of the bone and fracture site. **e–t** *see next page*

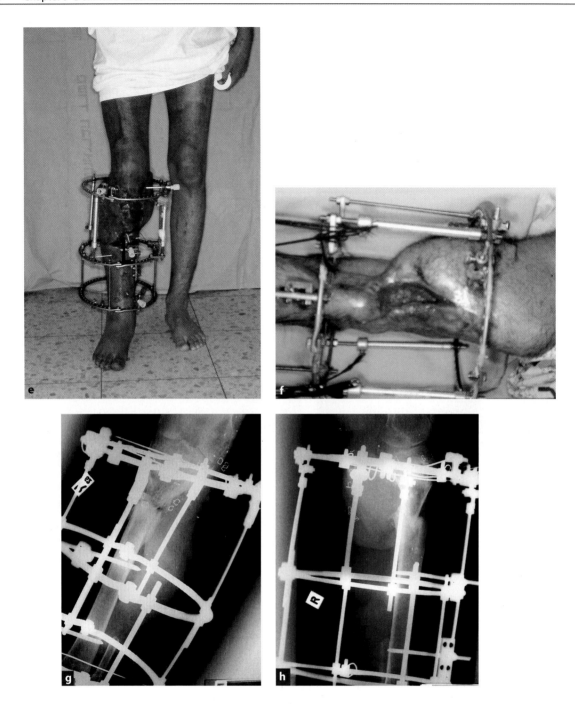

Fig. 3.3.1.1a–t. *(continued)* **e** Free tissue muscle latissimus dorsi flap and local muscle gastrocnemius flap were used to cover the exposed bone and fracture site. The unilateral tubular trans-knee frame was exchanged at this stage for a circular tibial Ilizarov frame with freeing of the knee joint. Clinical appearance showed complete soft-tissue coverage of the bone and fracture site. **f** Postoperative period was complicated by breaking of soft-tissue coverage, a septic wound over the proximal leg, and post-traumatic osteomyelitis of the tibial bone. Clinical appearance of the septic wound. **g,h** Repeated serial debridement of the fracture site with sequestrectomies was performed. Radiographs of tibial bone after sequestrectomy, shortening, and fixation in an external frame. **i–t** *see next page*

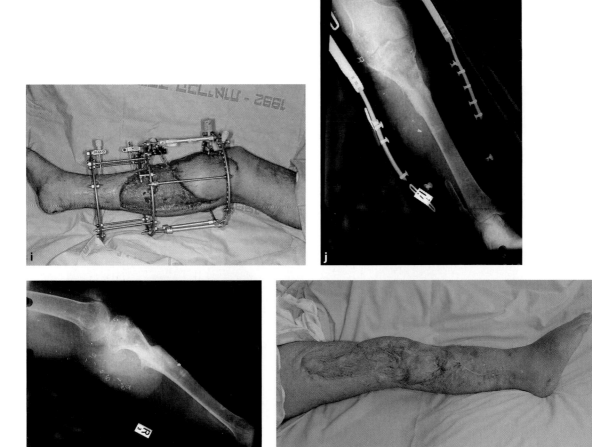

Fig. 3.3.1.1a–t. *(continued)* **i** Soft-tissue healing is achieved following radical sequestrectomy. Clinical appearance (medial view). **j,k** Long-duration local septic process and severe scarring in the fractures zone preclude a bone graft procedure to replace the tibial bone defect. Repeated cycles of distraction–compression in the external fixation frame were used to stimulate the bone regeneration process: 5 cm of bone regeneration was achieved. Radiographs 2 months after removing the Ilizarov frame demonstrate bone healing in good alignment with solid bone regeneration. Total time for external tibial fixation in the long-term treatment of this complex patient was 48 months. The patient was fully ambulatory during most of the treatment time. **l** Clinical photos at follow-up 5 years after removal of the Ilizarov frame demonstrate good function of the right lower limb. No recurrence of the local septic process was noted. **m–t** *see next page*

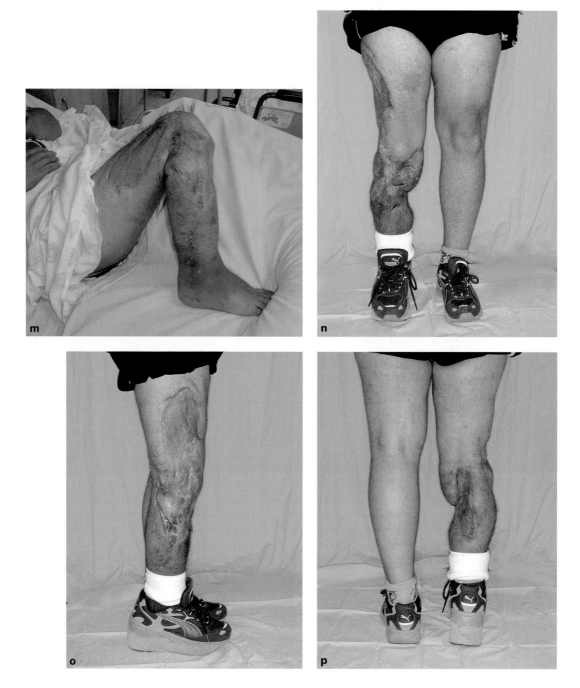

Fig. 3.3.1.1a–t. *(continued)* **m–p** Clinical photos at follow-up 5 years after removal of the Ilizarov frame demonstrate good function of the right lower limb. No recurrence of the local septic process was noted. **q–t** *see next page*

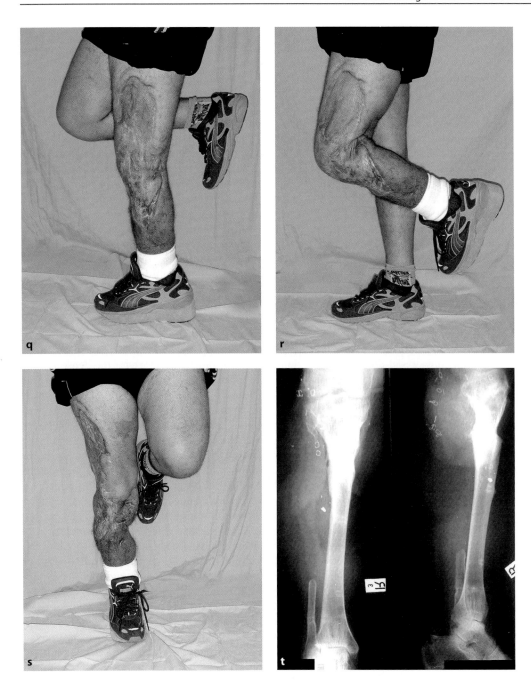

Fig. 3.3.1.1a–t. *(continued)* **q–s** Clinical photos at follow-up 5 years after removal of the Ilizarov frame demonstrate good function of the right lower limb. No recurrence of the local septic process was noted. **t** Radiograph examination at the 5-year follow-up demonstrates solid bone consolidation in good alignment. *Reproduced from Injury 36, Lerner et al Complications encountered while using thin-wire-hybrid-external fixation modular frames for fracture fixation, pp 590–598, © (2005), with permission from Elsevier [81]*

amount of heat generated during bone cutting procedures is a very significant factor, and the oscillating saw and Gigli saw techniques have some risk of thermal damage. Percutaneous minimally invasive techniques of subperiosteal bone cutting are preferable because only a small additional incision is required, and these procedures cause less damage to the tissues. The periosteum is incised longitudinally and elevated, using a small periosteal elevator. Multiple small 2-mm drill holes have to be made in the line of planned bone cutting to facilitate the procedure, and then the cortices are divided using a small 10-mm osteotome. Now, careful rotation of the rings in opposite directions until a cracking sound is heard should complete the procedure of bone division. In the next stage of the treatment, after a 7- to 10-day latency period, the original length of the bone shaft should be restored by slowly and gradually increasing the corticotomy gap and moving the intercalary segment away from the corticotomy site.

This technique permits not only consolidation of the fracture, but also the elimination of the bone defect by gradual controlled transfer of the mobilized intercalary bone fragment until its full contact and docking with the opposite bone fragment. Fixation in the external circular frame provides the necessary conditions for controlled gradual distraction in the zone of elongation and sufficient three-dimensional stability in the fracture zone by the simultaneous elimination of all types of deformities and providing needed effective compression in the fracture zone once the intercalary fragment has docked. This technique of reconstruction is usually indicated in the management of patients after high-energy shin fractures with severe tibial bone defects and intact fibular bone, when the length of the injured limb segment is safe. Reliable holding of the transported bone segment in the accurately assembled circular frame directs its controlled passage during the bone transport procedure. A rail technique of navigation of the bone fragment with introduction of a wire or thin nail into the medullary canal (often utilized in elective reconstructions) is unnecessary and bears the hazards of possible reactivation of infection and its extension along the nail and bone segment.

The procedure of distraction usually begins 7–10 days after performing the osteotomy/corticotomy. A distraction rate of 1 mm/day (0.25 mm q.i.d.) allows reconstruction of the bone loss. Restoration of extensive bone defects demands a long period of external fixation, including a period of distraction and maturation (approximately 1 month of distraction and external fixation per 1 cm of elongation). To shorten the length of the treatment, especially the external fixation time, a bifocal elongation osteotomy/corticotomy procedure may be performed.

Soft tissues lying in the route of the movement of the bone fragment (so-called bone transport) may shrink due to the absence of the inner hard tissue framework. This can result in a decrease of the diameter of the soft-tissue envelope. In these cases, if bone transport is continued, the skin can become invaginated on the upper end of the transported bone fragment. In addition, continuing the bone transport procedure can lead to compression and crushing of the indrawn skin between the bone fragments, creating atrophic disturbances in the skin due to its stretching and compression, even leading to skin thinning and denudation of the bone (Fig. 3.3.2.1).

With the onset of the signs of these dangerous complications, it is necessary to reduce the rate of bone fragment movement, or even to stop it completely. Reinforcement of the sagging tissues can be treated by the introduction of subcutaneous thin wires or by performing a special surgical procedure for the elevation of the sagged skin, using the translation of local soft-tissue flaps or excision of infolded skin.

A prolonged period, until bone contact in the fracture zone is achieved, may be needed when treating significant bone defects. Meanwhile, a dense fibrous scar may form near the target fragment, preventing intimate bone-to-bone contact and preventing bone union – the so-called docking problems. In these patients, an additional operative procedure to excise the dense fibrous tissues from the fracture site is needed to provide suitable conditions for bone contact. At the time of the debridement of the open trauma wound, it is desirable to perform an adjustment of the "kissing" frontal surfaces of the bone ends which are to meet after the transport later on, to improve their contact surfaces and to achieve better stability when compressive forces at the fracture site are applied during the final stage of transport. An optional cancellous autogenous bone graft can be added for the purpose of improving bone contact, and also for the filling of any residual defects on the frontal surfaces of the bone fragments. The bone grafting procedure can be done only on the condition that adequate coverage of the fracture zone exists and any signs of local infection are absent. Thus, using the bifocal technique, restoration of extensive bone loss can be performed without needing any massive bone grafting procedure.

A special technique is suitable for patients with open fractures and partial bone loss (where the bone defect does not involve the entire circumference of the injured bone). There remains a bone fragment (usually it is the posterior cortical area of the tibial bone), but one which is insufficient for achieving adequate bone stability due to its small size, even when bone union occurs. Moreover, such extant bone fragments do not permit the closure of the bone gap between the main fragments for achieving full bone contact, necessary for successful bone healing. Again, the local conditions of the soft tissues which have suffered from high-energy trauma exclude the use of an open bone graft replacement procedure to restore the lost bone. Controlled and gradual transfer of the bone fragment connected to the soft tissues, and corresponding to the frontal size to the bone defect, can be a suitable solution for this complex problem. This transferring

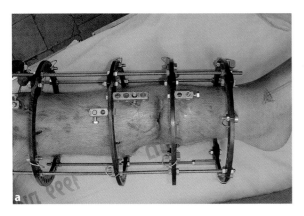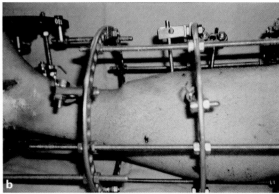

Fig. 3.3.2.1a,b. Clinical appearance of some soft-tissue problems during bone transport procedure. **a** Skin invagination at the "docking" site. **b** Severe skin tension over the sharp end of transported bone fragment

bone fragment can be detached from the frontal end of one of the main bone fragments (partial corticotomy with bone transport) (Fig. 3.3.2.2, Fig. 3.3.2.3).

3.3.3 Fibular Bone Translation, Foot Stabilization

In the treatment of patients with severe loss of tibial bone but where the fibular bone is essentially preserved, the choice of surgical procedure is especially difficult. Longitudinal splitting of the fibular bone in the area corresponding to the tibial bone defect and gradual translation of the split fibular fragment in a medial direction using Ilizarov principles is one option. Filling in by bone regeneration in the zone of fibular distraction can gradually replace a defect in the tibial bone. A bad general somatic or psychological condition, extensive complex trauma to soft tissues, and severe local scarring can contraindicate the use of this method and the traditional tibial bone transport method.

A technique of a single-stage translation of the fibular shaft to replace an absent tibial bone part is a suitable treatment option for these patients. This surgical procedure is less difficult to perform, demands less time and, most importantly, is significantly less traumatic in the treatment of these complex patients. With the advent of bone transport techniques, the use of the fibula to manage tibial defects has become less frequent [61]. Nevertheless, in some specific medical and social conditions, it may be a useful tool for limb salvage and reconstruction. It is very important to introduce a suitable end of the transferred bone fragment into the medullar canal of the corresponding tibial fragment. This can significantly increase stability of fixation and decrease the bone healing time. Fixation of the injured limb in the circular Ilizarov device allows holding of the transferred bone fragment with thin wires without massive

implanted devices of internal fixation. Furthermore, early controlled loading of the injured limb is possible in the three-dimensional stable fixation frame, as well as earlier loading of the transferred bone fragment, resulting in functional hypertrophy (Wolf's law) and bone healing (Fig. 3.3.3.1).

Expansion of the fixation frame to the foot can be used for more than stabilization of severe peri-articular injuries of the distal tibial bone. Including the foot in the tibial frame is a useful tool for severe hind-foot and mid-foot fractures, associated with tibial fractures. We recommend insertion of thin wires into the metatarsal and tarsal bones, and olive wires from both sides of the calcaneal bone to increase stability and diminish the possibility of pin-tract infection. A posteriorly placed threaded half-pin can also be used for fixation of calcaneal bone. Unstable fractures of the isolated medial or lateral ray of the foot can be fixed using a mini-external fixation set. This type of fixation preserves early motion in the tibio-talar and sub-talar joints. In addition, this type of fixator can be connected, if needed, to the proximally placed fixation system in the adjacent extremity segment (tibial fixation frame). A circular external fixator was reported as a useful tool in the treatment of complex calcaneal fractures with bone defects in blast mine injuries [43]. According to McHale and Gajewski [93], thin pin circular external fixation is a reasonable approach to the complex "floating ankle" pattern of injury in military personnel that results from blast injuries, especially in the presence of marked soft-tissue compromise (Fig. 3.3.3.2).

Metatarsal and toe fractures should be treated simultaneously using additional thin wire trans-fixation. These separate wires can be connected to the adjusting ring of the external fixation device to increase stability of fixation and avoid postoperative migration of thin wires.

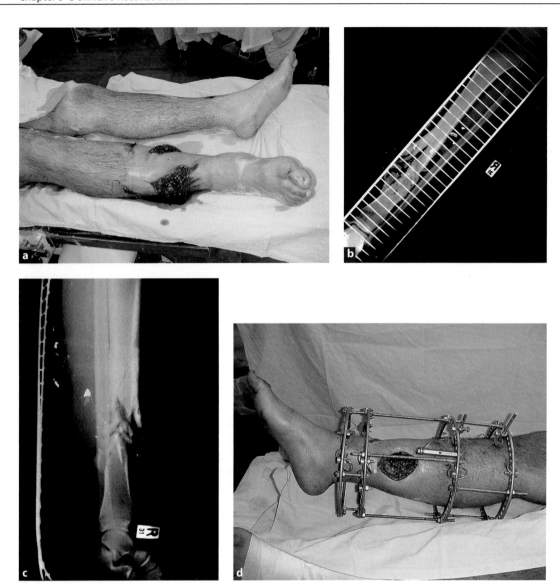

Fig. 3.3.2.2a–n. A 19-year-old male with open right tibial fracture Gustilo–Anderson type IIIC due to high-velocity gunshot injury. **a** Clinical appearance of right leg on admission, 1 h after battle trauma. **b,c** Radiographs on admission. Note bone comminuting with distal tibial loss. Radiological signs of foreign bodies in injury zone. **d** The patient had primary debridement of the wounds with vascular repair of the damage on two levels of the tibial posterior artery. Skeletal stabilization was performed using an Ilizarov circular frame. Clinical appearance of the leg after completing the operative procedure. **e–n** *see next page*

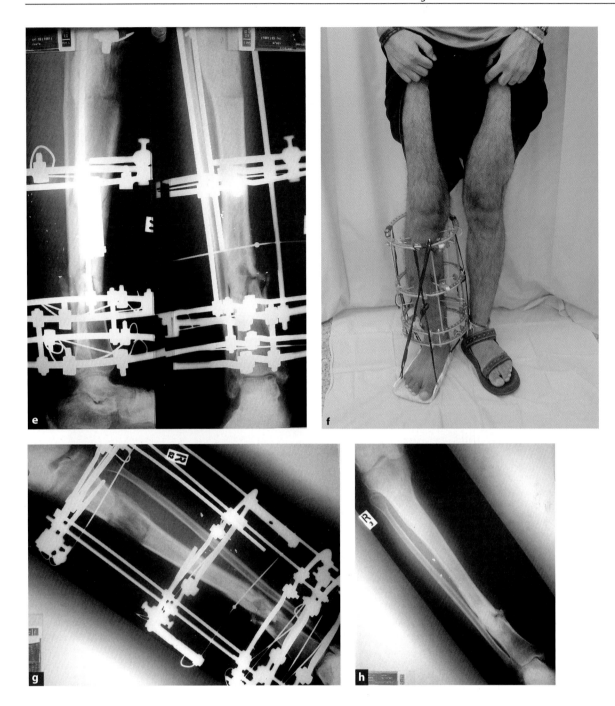

Fig. 3.3.2.2a–n. *(continued)* **e** Control postoperative radiograph of the leg. Note post-traumatic and post-debridement bone defect in the fracture zone. **f** Early full weight-bearing was allowed during the stabilization period in the external fixation frame. **g** Proximal tibial corticotomy was performed to eliminate the distal tibial bone defect using the bone transport technique. Radiological appearance of the bone regeneration 7 weeks after the corticotomy. **h** External frame was removed after 10 months of external fixation, followed by functional loading using a walking brace. Note radiological appearance of the solid bone consolidation. **i–n** *see next page*

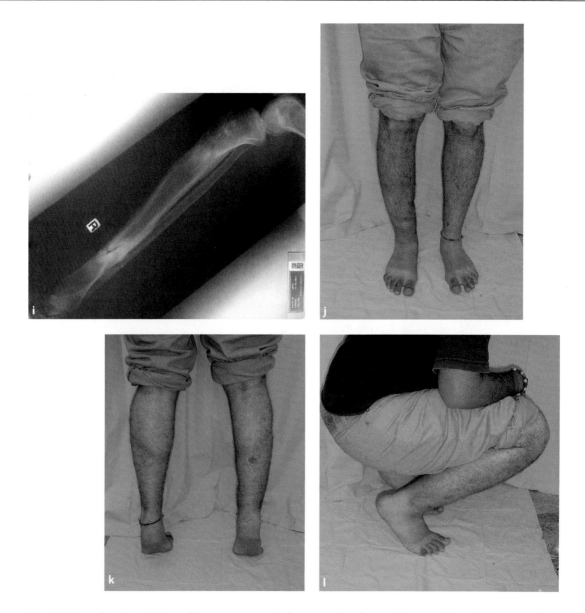

Fig. 3.3.2.2a–n. *(continued)* **i** External frame was removed after 10 months of external fixation, followed by functional loading using a walking brace. Note radiological appearance of the solid bone consolidation. **j–l** Clinical appearance on follow-up 12 months after removing the Ilizarov fixation frame. **m,n** *see next page*

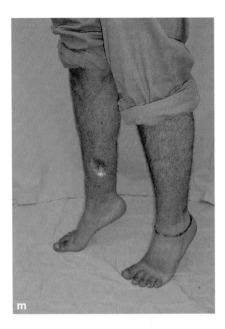
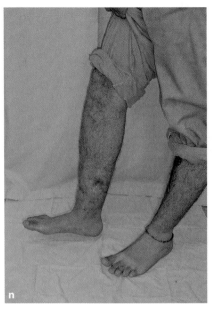

Fig. 3.3.2.2a–n. *(continued)* **m,n** Clinical appearance on follow-up 12 months after removing the Ilizarov fixation frame

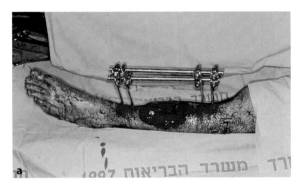
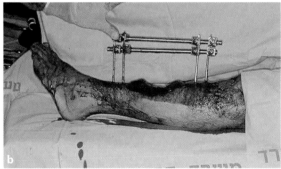

Fig. 3.3.2.3a–n. A 27-year-old male with open left tibial fracture Gustilo–Anderson type IIIB with soft-tissue and bone loss due to high-velocity gunshot injury. Primary debridement and stabilization using AO tubular external fixation frame were performed in another hospital. Five days later, he was referred to our hospital for surgical reconstruction. **a,b** Clinical appearance of left leg on admission. Skin and soft-tissue defect on anterior aspect of the leg. Fracture stabilization using AO unilateral tubular frame. **c–n** *see next page*

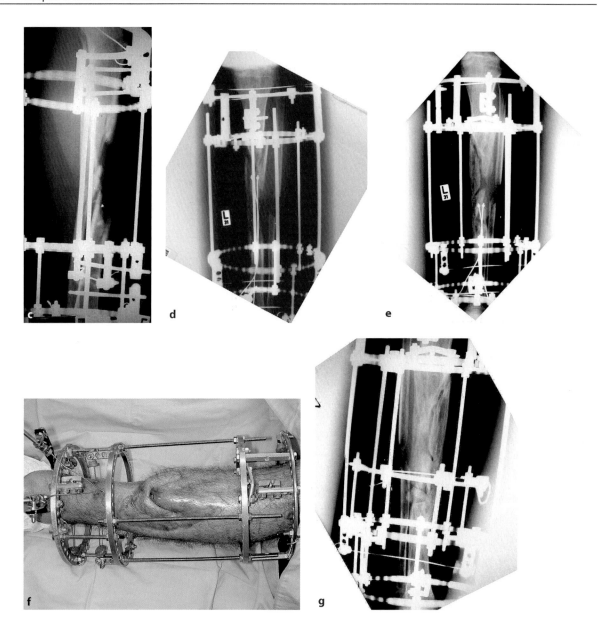

Fig. 3.3.2.3a–n. *(continued)* **c** Conversion of skeletal stabilization from a unilateral to an Ilizarov circular frame was performed. Control postoperative radiograph of the leg. Note bone comminuting with bone loss in the mid third of the tibia. **d,e** Proximal partial anterior tibial corticotomy was performed to eliminate the partial tibial bone defect by the bone transport technique using two crossed Kirschner wires. Radiological appearance of the two Kirschner wires with olives used for bone transport. **f** Bone transport process was complicated by skin invagination with trophic ulceration above the moved bone fragment. Clinical appearance of the skin invagination. Excision of the skin lesion, elimination of the invagination and closure of the wound by sutures were performed under local anesthesia. **g** Radiological appearance of maturation of bone regeneration after 6 weeks of bone transport. **h–n** *see next page*

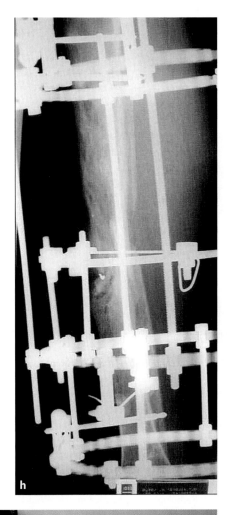

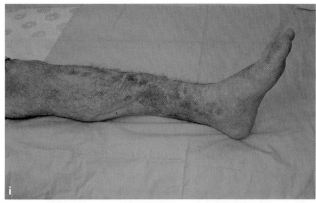

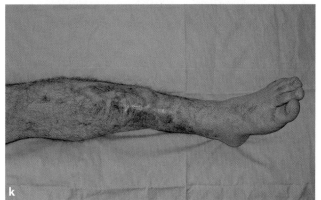

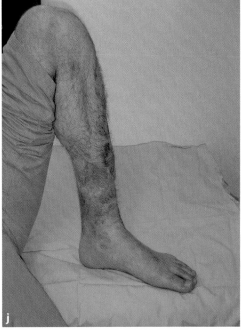

Fig. 3.3.2.3a–n. *(continued)* **h** Radiological appearance of the bone regeneration after completing the bone transport procedure. **i–k** External frame was removed after 10 months of external fixation. Clinical and radiological appearance 6 months after removing the Ilizarov external fixation frame. Solid bone consolidation is achieved in the fracture zone. Radiological signs of good bone regeneration. **l–n** *see next page*

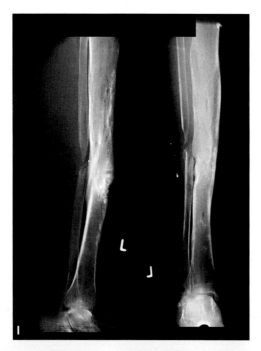

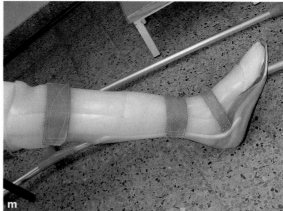

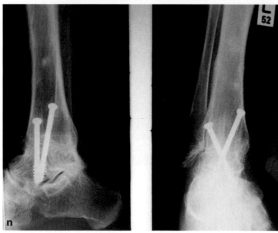

Fig. 3.3.2.3a–n. *(continued)* **l** External frame was removed after 10 months of external fixation. Clinical and radiological appearance 6 months after removing the Ilizarov external fixation frame. Solid bone consolidation is achieved in the fracture zone. Radiological signs of good bone regeneration. **m** Clinical appearance of post-traumatic drop foot due to severe damage to extensor muscle group. Functional loading is continued, using anti-drop-foot brace. **n** Tibio-talar arthrodesis using two crossed screws was performed to stabilize the ankle joint in the 90° position. Radiological appearance on follow-up 12 months later demonstrates solid tibio-talar bone fusion

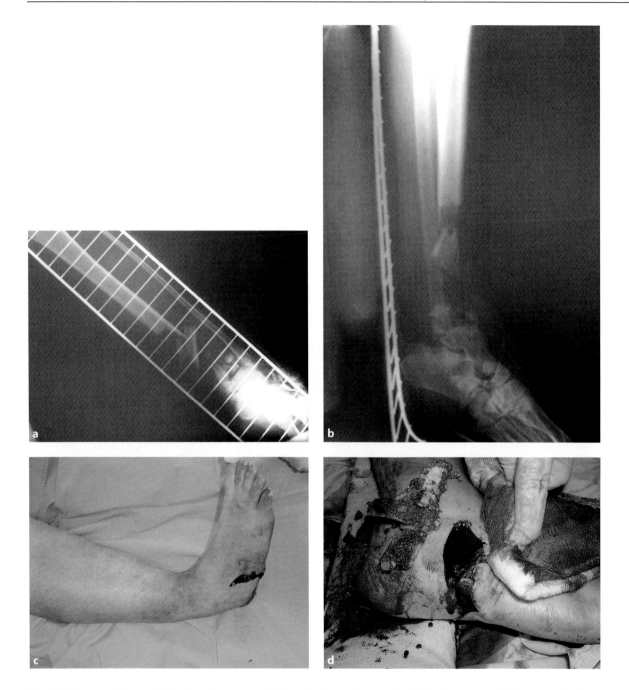

Fig. 3.3.3.1a–o. A 19-year-old female with an open right leg fracture and severe distal fibial loss due to a fall from an eight-floor building (suicide attempt). A time-consuming procedure of distraction osteogenesis was rejected as a suitable method of treatment due to the mental condition of this psychiatric patient. **a,b** Admission radiographs. Note bone comminuting with distal tibial loss. **c,d** Clinical appearance of right leg on admission. Note separated articular fragment of the distal tibial bone and severe varus deformity due to tibial bone loss. **e–o** *see next page*

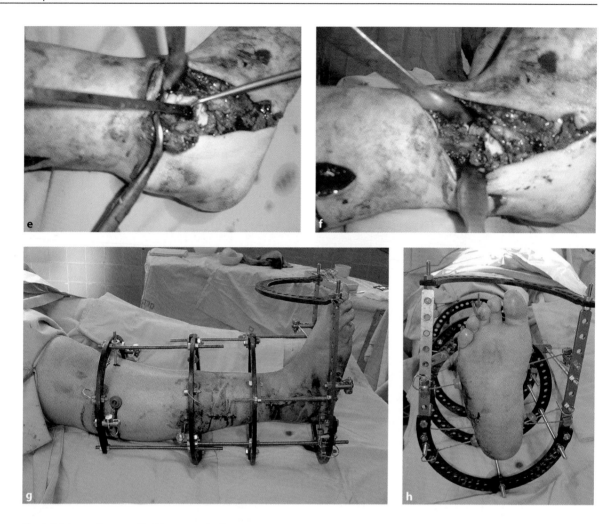

Fig. 3.3.3.1a–o. *(continued)* **e** The patient had primary debridement of the wound followed by acute medial translation of a distal fibular fragment to replace distal tibial loss. Clinical appearance of talus dome perforation in preparing the bone "bed" for the translated fibula. **f** Distal end of the fibular fragment was inserted into the prepared bone "bed." Proximal end of the fibular fragment was inserted into the tibial stump. **g,h** Clinical appearance of stabilization using Ilizarov external fixation frame. **i–o** *see next page*

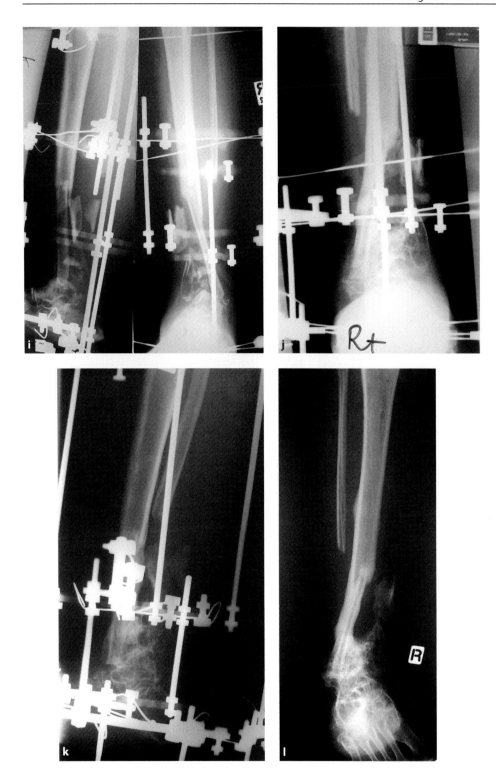

Fig. 3.3.3.1a–o. *(continued)* **i** Control radiograph after completing reconstructive procedure. Note the talar varus tilt on the antero-posterior film. **j,k** Additional close wedge osteotomy was performed to eliminate mal-alignment. **l** Full weight-bearing was allowed during the stabilization period in the external fixation frame. Solid bone consolidation was achieved after 6 months of Ilizarov fixation on both proximal and distal ends of the fibular graft. After removing the Ilizarov frame, functional loading was continued, using a walking brace. Note radiological appearance of functional hypertrophy of the loaded fibular bone fragment. **m–o** *see next page*

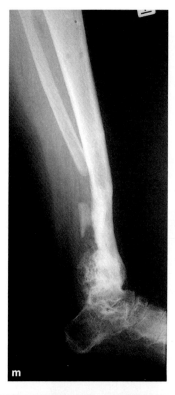

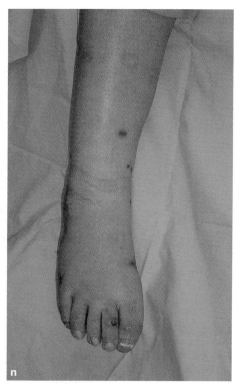

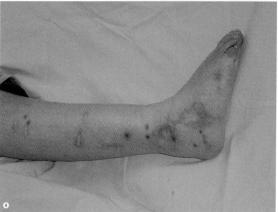

Fig. 3.3.3.1a–o. *(continued)* **m** Full weight-bearing was allowed during the stabilization period in the external fixation frame. Solid bone consolidation was achieved after 6 months of Ilizarov fixation on both proximal and distal ends of the fibular graft. After removing the Ilizarov frame, functional loading was continued, using a walking brace. Note radiological appearance of functional hypertrophy of the loaded fibular bone fragment. **n,o** Clinical appearance on follow-up 6 months after removing the Ilizarov fixation frame

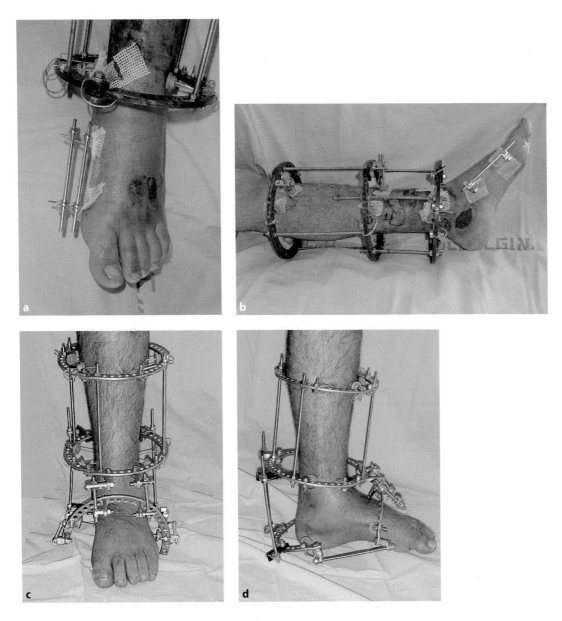

Fig. 3.3.3.2a–f. Clinical appearance of foot bone fractures using different external fixation frames. **a,b** Fixation of unstable fractures of the medial ray of the foot, using mini-external fixation set. **c,d** Using an Ilizarov tibial-foot frame for a calcaneal fracture, with closed reduction and external fixation. **e,f** *see next page*

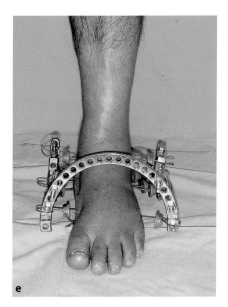
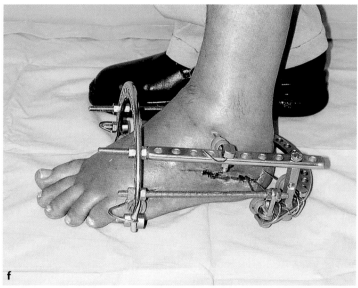

Fig. 3.3.3.2a–f. *(continued)* **e,f** Ilizarov frame for external fixation of mid-foot fracture. *Reprinted from Stein H et al. Minimally invasive surgical techniques for the reconstruction of calcaneal fractures. Orthopedics 2003; 26:1053–1056 with permission from SLACK Incorporated © [126]*

3.4 Acute Temporary Mal-Alignment in Limb Salvage

3.4.1 Acute Shortening

Open fractures cannot heal without good coverage of the fractured area, using well-vascularized soft tissue. Many complications can be avoided if this step is completed early. The soft-tissue reconstruction should eliminate any dead space. However, this step should be taken only when the debridement phase is completed.

The use of local and distant tissue flaps is not recommended for some patients due to the unavailability of local soft tissue or poor local potential of vascular supply (single vessel limb, conditions after re-vascularization procedures). According to Rozbruch et al. [111], revision flap coverage may not be an option after previous flap necrosis, and amputation remains the standard choice for such patients. For patients who suffered high-energy limb trauma which caused open fractures with extensive soft tissue and bone loss, we decided to apply the acute shortening technique, fixing the bone fragments using the Ilizarov external fixation device. Shortening of the severely injured limb can be used to facilitate closure of an extended soft-tissue defect. Soft-tissue coverage achieved by acute shortening decreases the need for local and distant tissue flaps and free tissue transfer. Acute shortening with subsequent progressive lengthening of the bone is an accepted alternative for patients with an absolute or relative contraindication for free and local flaps. Moreover, acute shortening of the bone allows

dealing with large soft-tissue and bone defects, eliminating the appearance of dead spaces at sites of tissue loss. Redundant soft tissue which results from an acute shortening procedure can be used to cover the exposed bone fragment and fracture area. This method may eliminate the need for long surgical procedures for soft-tissue and bone-length reconstructions. Complex and long procedures may be life-threatening for some patients with associated trauma of other organs. After applying the acute shortening procedure, the need for free flap reconstruction becomes rare, because most of the defects can be closed primarily or by using small local flaps and skin grafts. Moreover, acute shortening in the treatment of patients suffering from open fractures with vascular injuries (Gustilo type IIIC fractures) can eliminate the need for vascular grafting procedures, allowing end-to-end vascular suture even with the gap created by the debridement of the ends of the injured vessels.

For a transversely oriented soft-tissue defect, the acute shortening produces adequate contact of wound edges. In contrast, limb shortening for a longitudinally oriented wound can result in divergence of the wound edges, creating severe problems with closure of the soft-tissue defect. To take care of this problem, we use an S-shaped extension of the wound. This simple maneuver allows closure of the wound by counter transfer of the conformed skin-fascial flaps.

The Ilizarov technique with gradual distraction is not just a bone producer; soft tissue is gained as well. Progressive lengthening can be done, using either mono- or bi-focal techniques (Fig. 3.4.1.1).

In acute shortening, progressive lengthening using the Ilizarov device is based on the same principle of tension stress that allows bone regeneration. It is suggested that in these specific cases the lengthening phase can be started only after complete soft-tissue healing which, in our study, took 2–3 weeks. The gradual distraction rate provides acceptable cosmetic results and the bone length can be restored during the axial distraction for those with the bone edges that were well-approximated and aligned after the acute shortening. The callotasis technique has its limitation due to the restricted length that can be gained, mainly in the presence of extensive soft-tissue trauma caused by a high-energy injury. For these cases, an additional metaphyseal corticotomy/osteotomy was indicated. Two-level elongation corticotomy of the proximal and distal bone fragments is indicated for patients with extensive bone defects. This procedure improves the structural quality of the regenerated bone, while the elongation and fixation time is shortened.

Acute shortening of the upper limb is well tolerated by patients. The upper extremity is a non-weight-bearing organ and accepts shortening better, retaining more functions as compared to the lower limb during the drawn-out lengthening procedure. Temporary shortening of the severely injured limb after extensive radical debridement allows preservation of the potential for structural and functional restoration by guided graduated distraction with the Ilizarov method. The technique allows restoration of relatively large bone defects without the need for bone grafts and complicated local or free flaps, avoiding morbidity of donor sites and other serious complications. Additionally, the mechanical quality of the distracted bone is superior to cancellous bone grafts [79]. Lack of a donor site, morbidity, decreased operating time (important for patients with multiple organ trauma), good handling of both soft-tissue and bone defects, and low complication rates are the main advantages of acute shortening for complex limb injuries [79, 82, 111]. Bone defects and soft-tissue loss are handled simultaneously (Fig. 3.4.1.2).

3.4.2 Acute Shortening and Angulation

In a patient with combined bone and soft-tissue defects, it is mandatory to achieve skeletal stabilization and to cover the exposed bone as soon as possible, preferably during the initial care. However, in the treatment of some of these patients, especially those suffering from a one-sided large soft-tissue defect, the fracture site and bone remain uncovered even after completing acute shortening. Additional bone shortening is unacceptable. The only alternative for extensive tissue loss associated with bone exposure is soft-tissue reconstruction by a free flap. The presence of post-traumatic vessel disease [65], an entity described after trauma and including changes

in the vascular wall and the perivascular tissue, the bad general condition of the patient, and the absence of microsurgical skills reduce the chance of success of a free flap. Given these limited alternatives, acute shortening combined with angulation directed to the side of main soft-tissue loss to cover the exposed bone appears to be the accepted treatment choice, diminishing the soft-tissue defect [82]. In this way, further shortening of the bone or the use of complicated soft-tissue reconstructive procedures can be avoided. Primary closure of the soft-tissue defect can be achieved without tension on the edges of the wound. The peripheral pulses, the color, and capillary refilling must be checked at this stage to verify that there is no vascular compromise. The acute angulation must be stopped if these indices worsen during the manipulation. Continuous monitoring of the circulation in the distal segments of the operated limb must be performed. For this reason we perform this procedure without draping the foot or hand.

The angulated bone fragments are fixed using a hinged Ilizarov fixation frame. The hinges above the angulation place must be locked (Fig. 3.4.2.1).

The gradual progressive correction of mal-angulation can be initiated only when the wound is completely closed, usually 3–4 weeks after the angulation procedure. The Ilizarov external fixator gains soft-tissue length by stretching the skin and the scars, resulting in a good soft-tissue envelope at the end of bone distraction. The pace of correction depends on the scar and soft-tissue condition. Any haste in the commencement and progression of this procedure must be avoided! When re-alignment is achieved, an elongation corticotomy can be performed (proximally or distally – according to the local tissue conditions and location of the longest bone fragment). In patients with large bone defects, a second corticotomy can be performed to increase the rate of lengthening [82]. Full weight-bearing can be allowed in the early postoperative period, attaching an additional foot ring or plate to the external fixation frame, according to the relative shortening created. Intensive daily physiotherapy for muscle strengthening and prevention of muscle stiffness and joint contractures starts on the first postoperative day and must be continued during the entire fixation period (Fig. 3.4.2.2, Fig. 3.4.2.3, Fig. 3.4.2.4).

3.4.3 Acute Shortening, Angulation, and Malrotation

Even after acute shortening and angulation in treating one 49-year-old patient who suffered from an open Gustilo type IIIC distal tibial fracture with severe tissue loss, the antero-medial side of the tibial bone and fracture site remained uncovered with a 7 cm × 3 cm soft-tissue defect. An additional malrotation of the foot and distal tibial fragment can result in a decrease of the

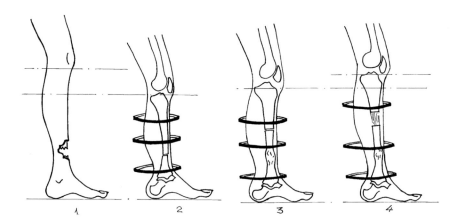

Fig. 3.4.1.1. Schematic representation of temporary acute shortening technique. *1* Presentation of the limb on admission – open fracture with bone and soft tissue loss. *2* Debridement with acute shortening and stabilization in the external circular frame. *3* Proximal elongation tibial osteotomy is performed. *4* Limb length is restored by bone regeneration in the osteotomy site

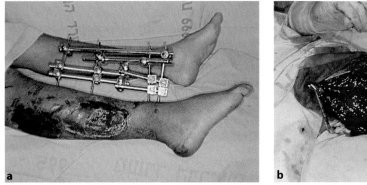
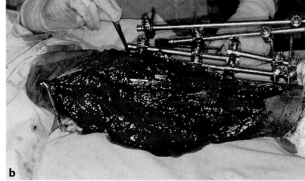

Fig. 3.4.1.2a–n. A 19-year old male with crush injury to the left lower limb and open comminuted tibial fracture due to road traffic accident (the leg was crushed under a weight of about 500 kg for more than 30 min). Primary debridement of the wound was followed by unilateral external fixation for tibial fracture stabilization. On the 5th day post-trauma, the skin and soft tissue became necrotic and the patient was returned to the operating room for a repeat debridement procedure. **a** Clinical appearance of the leg on the 5th day after trauma. Note necrotic findings on the skin and soft tissues, but the true extent of the soft-tissue injury is not apparent. **b** Clinical photo of large soft-tissue defect after performing surgical exploration and repeated extensive debridement of all necrotic soft tissues, and also denuded and comminuted bone fragments with questionable viability. **c–n** *see next page*

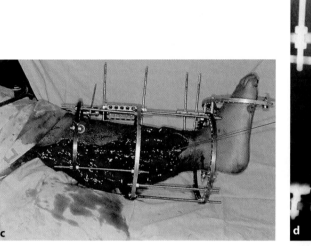

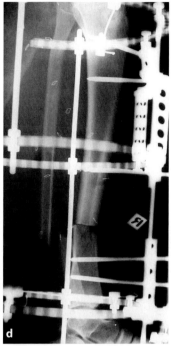

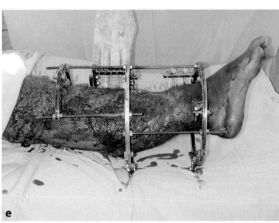

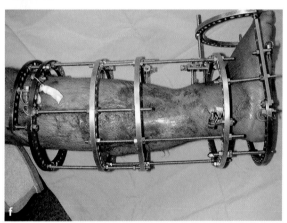

Fig. 3.4.1.2a–n. *(continued)* c Completing the debridement procedure, acute tibial shortening was performed, with conversion of unilateral external fixator to the circular Ilizarov frame. d Radiograph after completing the bone debridement, acute 8-cm shortening and external fixation by Ilizarov frame. e Clinical appearance 3 weeks after trauma. Good skin graft healing on all surfaces of the wound. f Re-montage of the Ilizarov frame and proximal tibial corticotomy for limb length restoration were performed 30 days after trauma. Note the foot attachments to the tibial external fixation frame for temporarily keeping the foot in a 90° position during the elongation period to avoid equinus deformity. **g–n** *see next page*

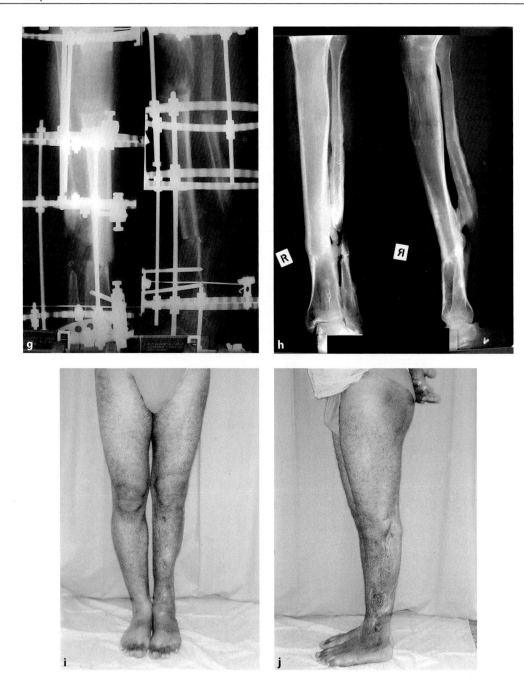

Fig. 3.4.1.2a–n. *(continued)* **g** Ilizarov external fixation 3 months later. Radiological appearance of good bone regeneration. **h** Total time of external tibial fixation – 10 months. Radiological photos show bone consolidation of the tibial fracture, solid bone regeneration after completing 8-cm tibial elongation. **i,j** Clinical photos at follow-up 2 years after removal of the Ilizarov frame. **k–n** *see next page*

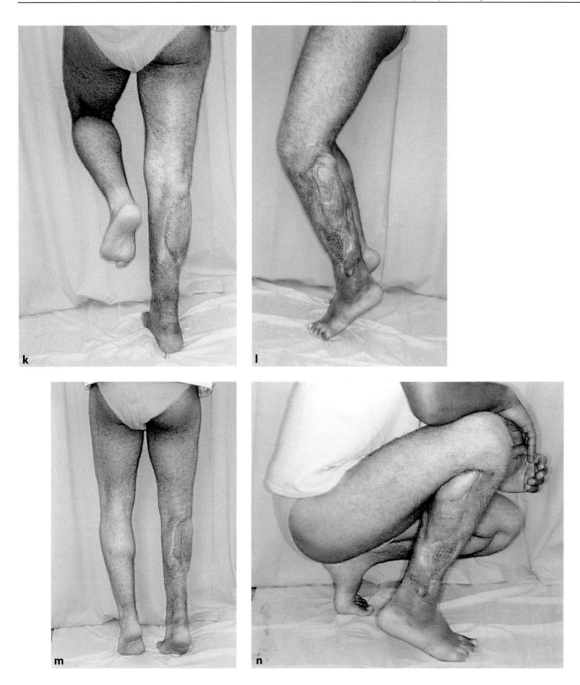

Fig. 3.4.1.2a–n. *(continued)* **k–n** Clinical photos at follow-up 2 years after removal of the Ilizarov frame. **c,d,f,g** *Reproduced with permission from © Lippincott Williams and Wilkins Lerner et al (2004) Acute shortening – modular treatment modality for severe combined bone and soft tissue loss of the extremities. J Trauma 57:603–608 [79]*

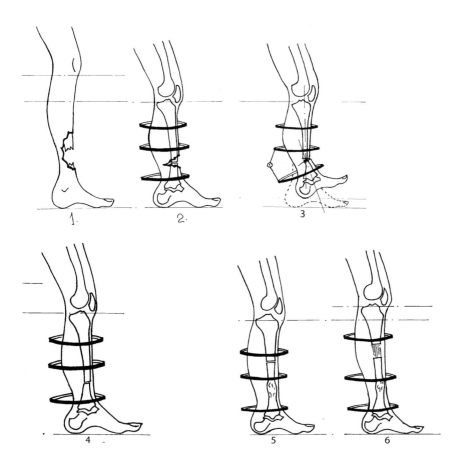

Fig. 3.4.2.1. Schematic representation of technique of temporary acute shortening and angulation. *1* Presentation of the limb on admission – open fracture with bone and soft-tissue loss. *2* Debridement with acute shortening and stabilization in the external circular frame. Note uncovered fracture site after performing shortening procedure. *3* Acute angulation is performed to diminish the soft-tissue wound and coverage of the fracture site. *4* The leg is gradually re-aligned using the Ilizarov frame. *5* Proximal elongation tibial steotomy is performed. *6* Limb length is restored by bone regeneration in the osteotomy site

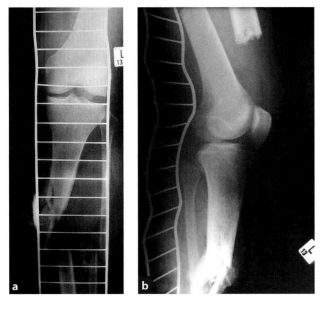

Fig. 3.4.2.2a–z4. A 22-year-old male. This victim of a motorcycle accident was referred to us 2 weeks after he sustained a left Gustilo–Anderson IIIB open tibial fracture and an ipsilateral closed femoral fracture. The patient had primary debridement of the wounds followed by unilateral external fixation for femoral and tibial fracture stabilization. The tibial fracture became infected and the patient was referred to us. **a–b** Initial radiographs of left femur and tibia demonstrate "floating knee" with displaced femoral shaft fracture and displaced comminuted tibial fracture with bone loss. **c–z4** *see next page*

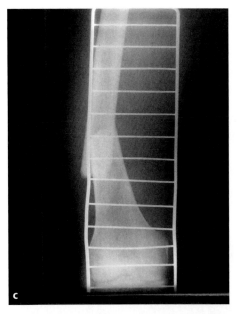
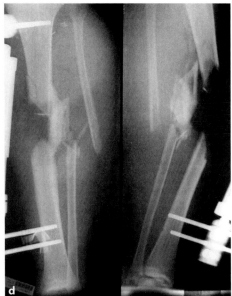

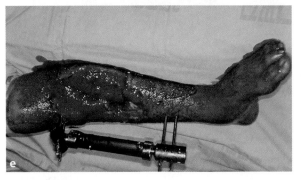
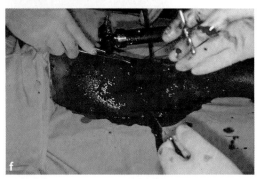

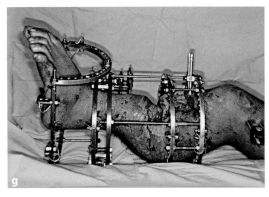
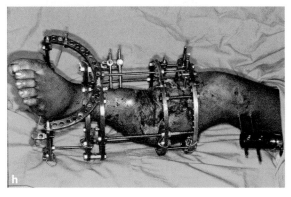

Fig. 3.4.2.2a–z4. *(continued)* **c** Initial radiographs of left femur and tibia demonstrate "floating knee" with displaced femoral shaft fracture and displaced comminuted tibial fracture with bone loss. **d** Radiograph of the leg on admission. Note the displaced comminuted tibia-fibula fracture with bone loss. **e** The clinical photo shows the infected wound with soft-tissue defect on admission. **f** Clinical photo of surgical exploration and repeated debridement of necrotic soft tissue and bone on admission. Gigly saw is used for resection of necrotic tibial fragments. After complete removal of all necrotic bone, the remaining tibial defect was 22 cm long. **g,h** After completing the debridement procedure, acute tibial shortening was performed to simultaneous correct the large bone and soft-tissue defects. External fixation in the circular Ilizarov frame is performed. Note that although the bone gap was closed at the end of the shortening procedure, the anterior aspect of the fracture was still open. **i–z4** *see next page*

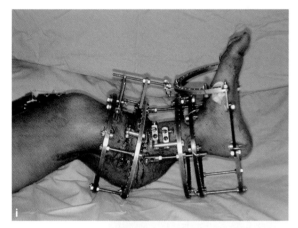

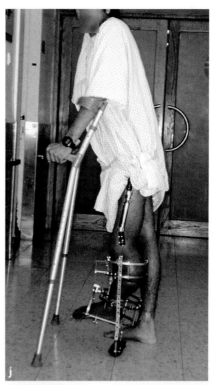

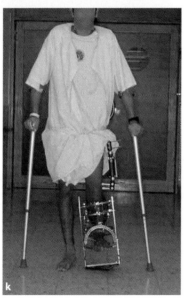

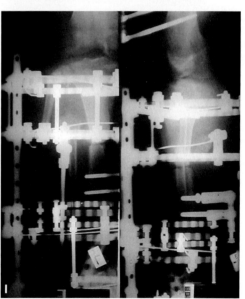

Fig. 3.4.2.2a–z4. *(continued)* **i** Combining shortening with a 50° anterior angulation is used to close the wound at the exposed tibia and fracture sites. The angulated bone fragments are secured with a hinged Ilizarov frame. **j,k** Partial weight-bearing on the left lower limb 3 weeks after admission. **l** Three weeks after the angulation procedure, the wounds were completely closed and progressive correction of the angulation was initiated. Three weeks later, the mal-alignment was gradually restored (clinical and radiological views) and compression of the tibial bone fragments was performed. Note the additional attachments to the external fixation frame for temporary compensation of the lower limb length discrepancy and performing weight-bearing on the injured limb. **m–z4** *see next page*

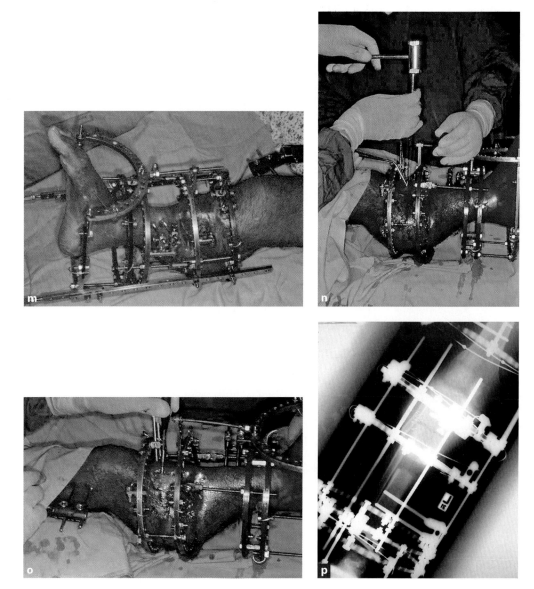

Fig. 3.4.2.2a–z4. *(continued)* **m** Three weeks after the angulation procedure, the wounds were completely closed and progressive correction of the angulation was initiated. Three weeks later, the mal-alignment was gradually restored (clinical and radiological views) and compression of the tibial bone fragments was performed. Note the additional attachments to the external fixation frame for temporary compensation of the lower limb length discrepancy and performing weight-bearing on the injured limb. **n,o** Clinical photos of proximal tibial corticotomy using a small osteotome for bone elongation. **p** Distraction was started 7 days later at a rate of 0.25 mm q.i.d. **q–z4** *see next page*

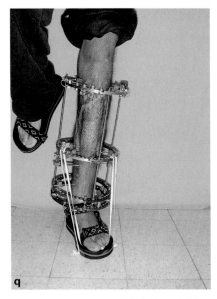

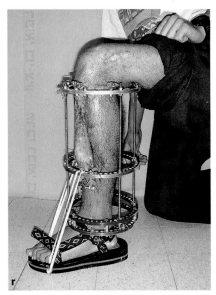

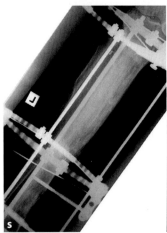

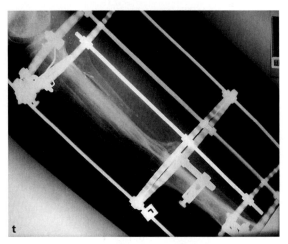

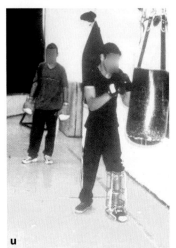

Fig. 3.4.2.2a–z4. *(continued)* **q–t** Due to the large bone defect (22 cm), a second corticotomy in the distal part of the tibia was performed to increase the rate of lengthening (80 days later). At this stage, the femoral unilateral external fixator was exchanged for an Ilizarov frame to gain more stability for the femoral fracture. The distraction on the distal tibial corticotomy site was initiated at a rate of 0.25 mm t.i.d. After about 3 months of bi-level distraction at a rate 1.75 mm a day, the tibia had regained its original length (clinical and radiological views). **u** Clinical photos of full physical activity during external fixation period, including contact sports and swimming. **v–z4** *see next page*

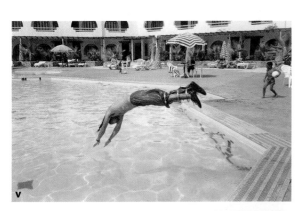

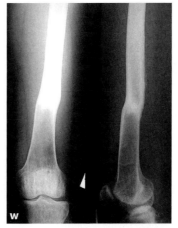

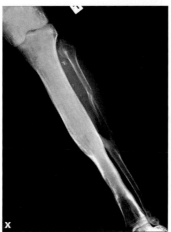

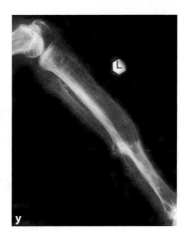

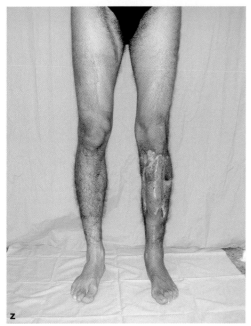

Fig. 3.4.2.2a–z4. *(continued)* **v** Clinical photos of full physical activity during external fixation period, including contact sports and swimming. **w–y** Total time of external femoral fixation: 223 days; external tibial fixation: 371 days. Radiographs show bone consolidation of both femoral and tibial fractures, solid bone regeneration after completing bi-level 22-cm tibial elongation. **z** Clinical photo at follow-up 1 year after removal of the Ilizarov frame. Examination of the left knee and ankle joints demonstrated painless and nearly full active and passive range of movements. **z1–z4** *see next page*

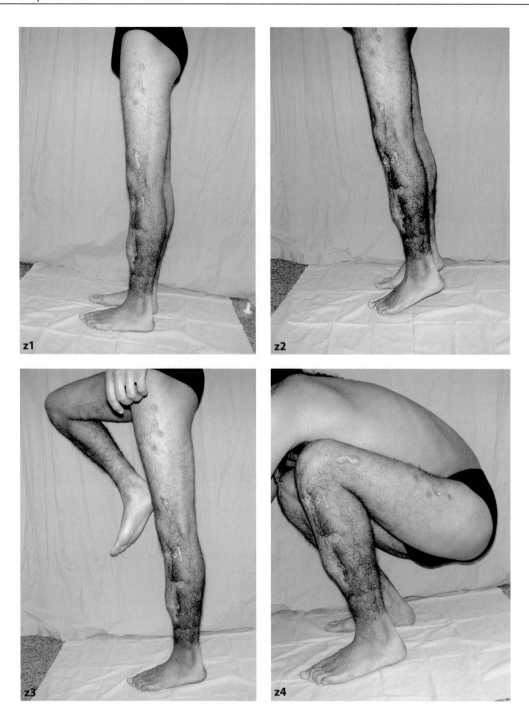

Fig. 3.4.2.2a–z4. *(continued)* **z1–z4** Clinical photo at follow-up 1 year after removal of the Ilizarov frame. Examination of the left knee and ankle joints demonstrated painless and nearly full active and passive range of movements. **a,e,i,s** *Reprinted from Current Orthopaedics 15, Stein H, Lerner A Advances in the treatment of chronic osteomyelitis, pp 451–456, © (2001), with permission from Elsevier [123].* **d,e,j,q,x,z1,z4** *Reproduced with permission from © Lippincott Williams and Wilkins; Lerner et al (2005) Unilateral, hinged external fixation frame for elbow compression arthrodesis: the stepwise attainment of a stable 90-degree flexion position. A case report. J Orthop Trauma 19:52–55 [83]*

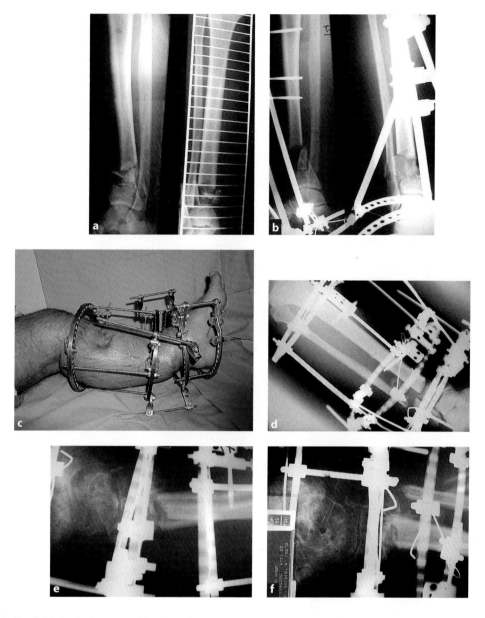

Fig. 3.4.2.3a–k. A 59-year-old male with open comminuted distal tibial fracture Gustilo–Anderson type IIIB with soft-tissue loss on the anterior aspect of the leg due to a road traffic accident. **a** Radiograph on admission. **b** Surgical debridement was performed. The realigned fracture was fixed using a trans-ankle hybrid external fixation frame. **c** Seven days after the trauma, a repeated surgical debridement with necrectomy and removal of free bone fragments was performed. To minimize the bone debridement and the soft-tissue defect and to compact the bone edges, acute shortening (6 cm) and additional anterior 40° angulation at the fracture site were completed. The angulated bone fragments were secured with a hinged Ilizarov frame (clinical photo). **d,e** Three weeks later, after healing of the wounds on the anterior aspects of the legs, gradual correction of misalignment was started. The axial alignment was restored over a period of about 3 weeks, by performing isolated anterior distraction of the hinged external fixation frame (radiograph). **f** Radiological photos 4 months after surgery show process of consolidation. Proximal corticotomy for elongation and length restoration was rejected by the patient. Seven months after the trauma, the Ilizarov frame was removed. **g–k** *see next page*

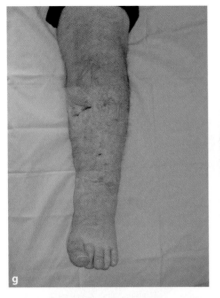

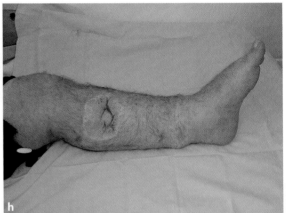

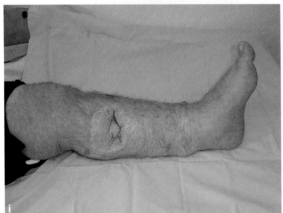

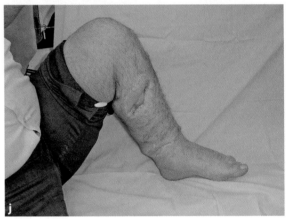

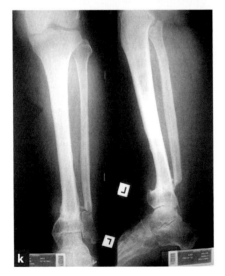

Fig. 3.4.2.3a–k. *(continued)* **g–k** Follow-up after 12 months. Clinical and radiological views

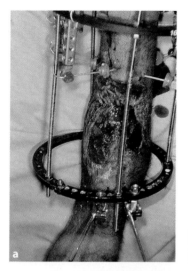

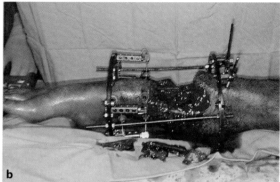

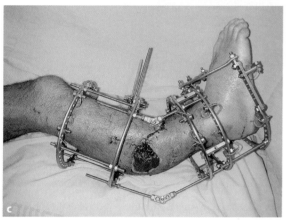

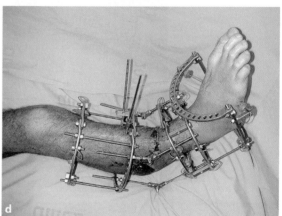

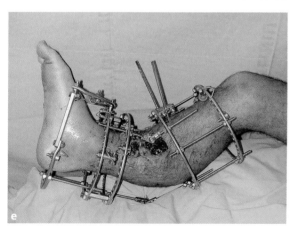

Fig. 3.4.2.4a–p. A 33-year-old male. In a road traffic accident, he sustained a left Gustilo–Anderson IIIB open right tibial fracture with anterior soft-tissue loss. The patient had debridement of the wounds followed by circular external fixation for primary tibial fracture stabilization. **a** Clinical view 1 week later. Circular external fixation with appearance of necrotic changes in the wound. **b** Surgical debridement was repeated and removal of necrotic soft tissue and some free tibial fragments was performed, leaving a bony gap of 13 cm. **c–e** Completing the debridement procedure, combining of shortening with a 50° anterior angulation was performed to close the wound on the exposed tibia and fracture sites. The angulated bone fragments were secured with a hinged Ilizarov frame. **f–p** *see next page*

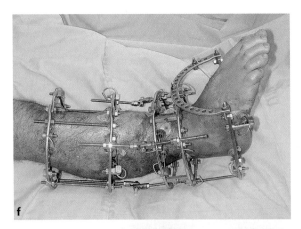

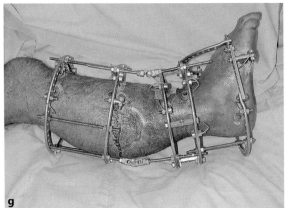

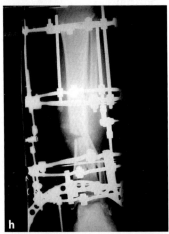

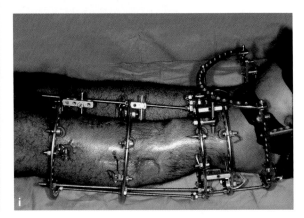

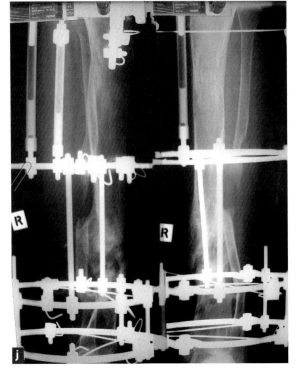

Fig. 3.4.2.4a–p. *(continued)* **f,g** Three weeks after the angulation procedure, the wounds were completely closed and progressive correction of the angulation was initiated. Clinical photo 2 weeks later shows partial correction of mal-angulation. **h** Three weeks later, the mal-alignment was gradually restored (radiological views) and compression of the tibial bone fragments was carried out. **i,j** Proximal tibial corticotomy for elongation was performed. The limb was distracted at a rate of 0.25 mm q.i.d. After 4 months of distraction, the tibia had regained its original length (clinical and radiological views). **k–p** *see next page*

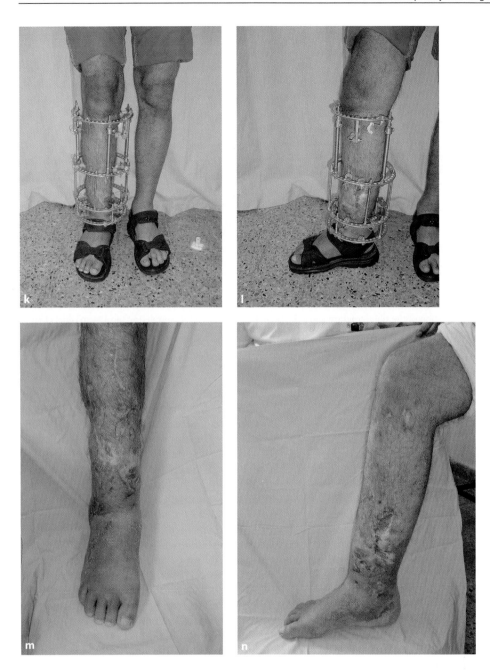

Fig. 3.4.2.4a–p. *(continued)* **k,l** Clinical view shows freeing of ankle joint after completing the bone elongation process and full weight-bearing during the external fixation period. **m–n** Clinical and radiological photos at follow-up 1 year after removal of the Ilizarov frame. Radiological photos demonstrate bone consolidation of the tibial fracture and solid bone regeneration after completing the 13-cm tibial elongation. **o,p** *see next page*

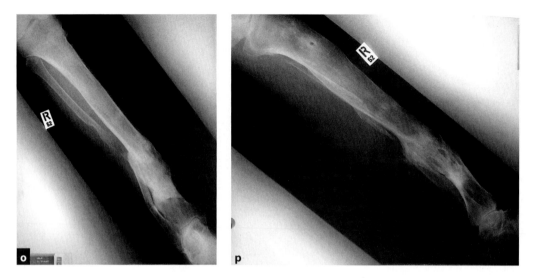

Fig. 3.4.2.4a–p. *(continued)* **o,p** Clinical and radiological photos at follow-up 1 year after removal of the Ilizarov frame. Radiological photos demonstrate bone consolidation of the tibial fracture and solid bone regeneration after completing the 13-cm tibial elongation

wound size, bringing its edges together. This additional procedure allowed the coverage of the fracture site. Gradual derotation of the limb in the Ilizarov frame was performed later, together with distraction of the bone regenerate and limb length restoration.

Important: the fixed limb segment is usually eccentrically situated in the circular fixation frame, and within the limb segment the bone itself is also eccentrically located. Remember that the rotation center of the frame in performing the rotation motion is always placed exactly in the center of the ring. Thus, performing rotation in the circular frame, a bone fragment, attached in an eccentric position into the ring (outside the center of rotation), can result in lateral displacement with regard to the bone fragment, fixed on the opposite site of the external fixation frame. The greater the malrotation, the more asymmetric is the position occupied by the bone fragments in the rings, and the greater is the lateral translation of the fragments in the final stage of the derotation procedure. By attaching additional connection plates to the ring at the point nearest to the bone, the external configuration

of the frame is changed. In this way the bone is placed in the central position of the modified external frame and also in the center of rotation. In this way, the bone will retain its central position during the process of derotation and lateral displacement can be avoided (Fig. 3.4.3.1).

Continuing the treatment of this complex patient, gradual derotation of the limb in the Ilizarov frame was performed later, together with distraction of the bone regenerate and limb length restoration. The derotation process can be combined in time with the process of elongation in the frame, which can significantly shorten the general duration of external fixation time and, accordingly, the general treatment time (Fig. 3.4.3.2).

In conclusion, temporary malpositioning of the segments (shortening, mal-angulation, and malrotation) with subsequent gradual correction of misalignment avoids extensive bone resection in patients with large soft-tissue defects. The stable three-dimensional bone stabilization in the circular fixation frame allows early functional weight-bearing even in such complex patients.

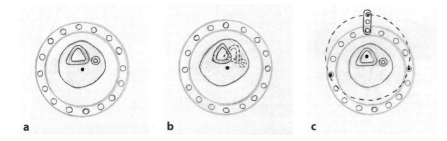

Fig. 3.4.3.1a–c. Plane of derotation in the circular fixation frame. **a** Note eccentric position of fixed segment of the limb and also bone fragments in the circular fixation frame. Rotation center of the frame in performing the rotation motion placed in the center of the ring. **b** Lateral displacement of the eccentrically placed bone fragment due to rotation in the circular frame. **c** Attachment of additional connection plates helps to change external configuration of the frame. Resulting from this procedure, the bone placed in the central position of the external frame is also in the center of rotation

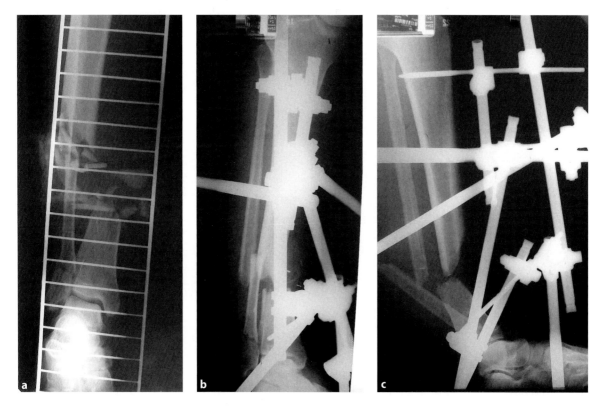

Fig. 3.4.3.2a–z5. A 49-year-old male who suffered from open Gustilo type IIIC left distal tibial fracture with severe tissue and bone loss due to a road traffic accident. Lesion of tibialis anterior and posterior arteries was found on exploration of the wound. **a** Radiograph at time of injury. **b,c** Primary emergency care was carried out with debridement of soft tissues, repair of tibialis anterior and posterior arteries, and stabilization of the fracture with a tubular external fixator. Fixation of bone fragments was performed with antero-medial angulation due to severe soft-tissue loss on the antero-medial side of the tibial bone and fracture site. **d–z5** *see next page*

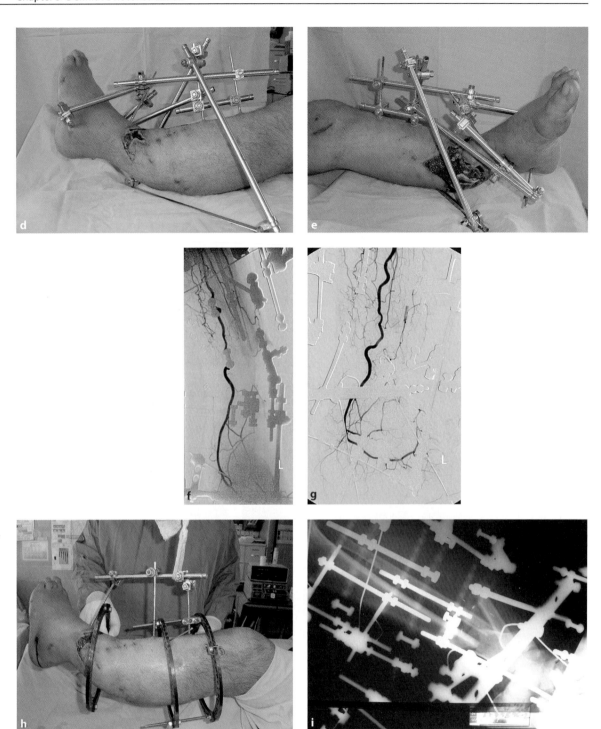

Fig. 3.4.3.2a–z5. *(continued)* **d,e** Even after performing antero-medial angulation, the fracture site remained uncovered, with a 7 cm × 3 cm soft-tissue defect. **f,g** Angiography performed in planning the definitive reconstructive procedure shows occlusion of the repaired tibialis anterior artery. **h** Assembly of a circular Ilizarov external fixator was performed, preserving the position of the bone fragments achieved by the primary fixation procedure (note the fixation of cantilevered half-pins of the primary tubular fixator to the rings of the Ilizarov frame). Thus, the site of vascular anastomosis of the single remaining repaired tibialis posterior artery was undisturbed. **i** Additional malrotation of foot and distal tibial fragment resulted in a significant decrease of wound width, bringing its edges together. Radiological and clinical views of the mal-aligned limb included acute shortening, angulation, and malrotation. The angulated bone fragments were secured with a hinged Ilizarov frame, included foot attachment. **j–z5** *see next page*

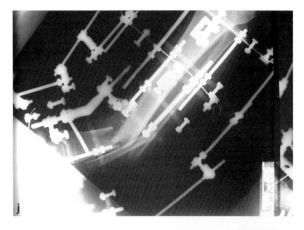

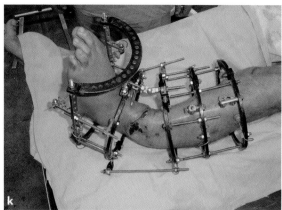

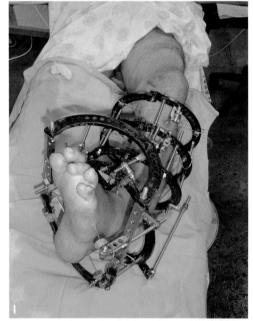

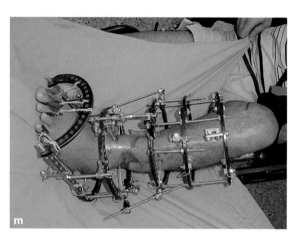

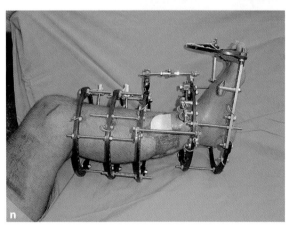

Fig. 3.4.3.2a–z5. *(continued)* **j–l** Additional malrotation of foot and distal tibial fragment resulted in a significant decrease of wound width, bringing its edges together. Radiological and clinical views of the mal-aligned limb included acute shortening, angulation, and malrotation. The angulated bone fragments were secured with a hinged Ilizarov frame, included foot attachment. **m,n** Four weeks after the angulation procedure, the wound was completely closed and progressive correction of the angulation was initiated. Three weeks later, the angular mal-alignment was gradually restored (clinical and radiological views) and compression of the tibial bone fragments was performed. **o–z5** *see next page*

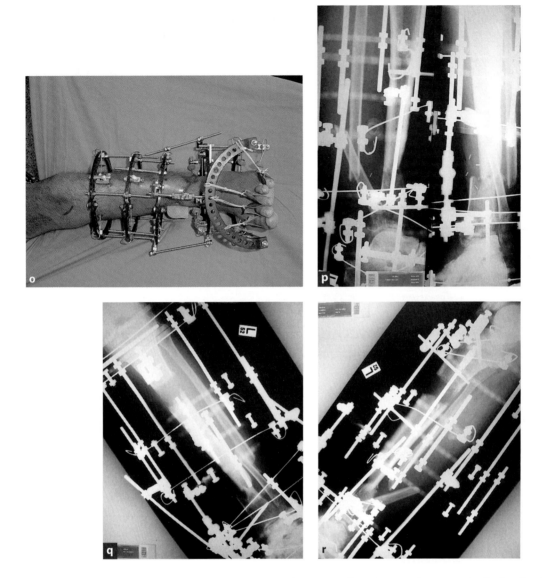

Fig. 3.4.3.2a–z5. *(continued)* **o,p** Four weeks after the angulation procedure, the wound was completely closed and progressive correction of the angulation was initiated. Three weeks later, the angular mal-alignment was gradually restored (clinical and radiological views) and compression of the tibial bone fragments was performed. **q,r** Radiological photos taken 2 months after proximal elongation tibial corticotomy show good bone regeneration. **s–z5** *see next page*

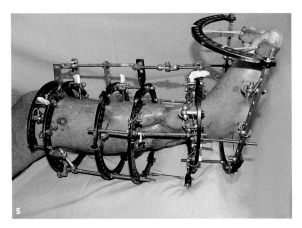

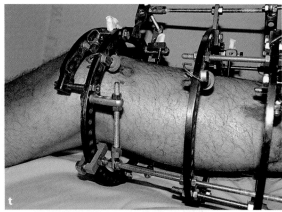

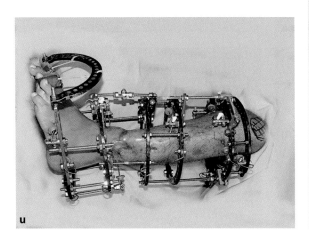

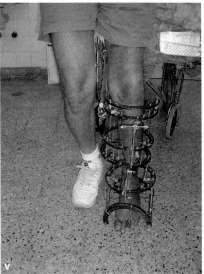

Fig. 3.4.3.2a–z5. *(continued)* **s–u** Note attachment of additional connection plates to the ring changes the external configuration of the frame. Thus, during the derotation process the bone retains its central position, and lateral displacement can be avoided. **v** Full weight-bearing on the fixed Ilizarov frame leg at an early stage of the derotation procedure. **w–z5** *see next page*

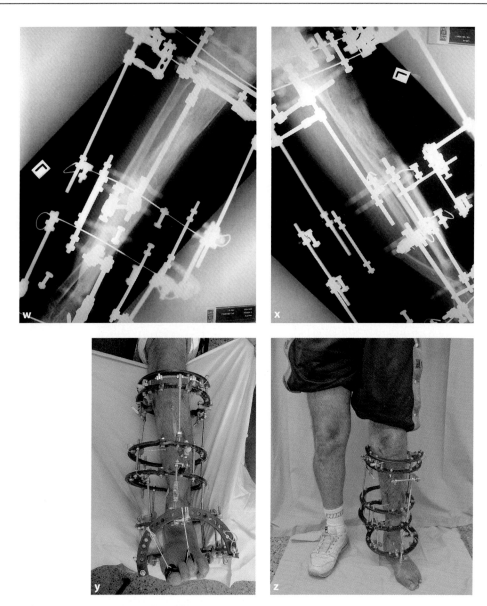

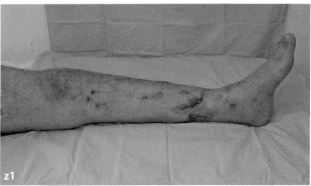

Fig. 3.4.3.2a–z5. *(continued)* **w–z** Clinical and radiological photos after completing the reconstruction procedure. A 12-cm elongation was achieved and leg length was restored. Total time in external tibial fixation: 13 months. **z1** Clinical and radiological photos at follow-up 6 months after removal of the Ilizarov frame. Radiological photos demonstrate bone consolidation of the distal tibial fracture, with solid bone regeneration after completing a 12-cm proximal tibial elongation. **z2–z5** *see next page*

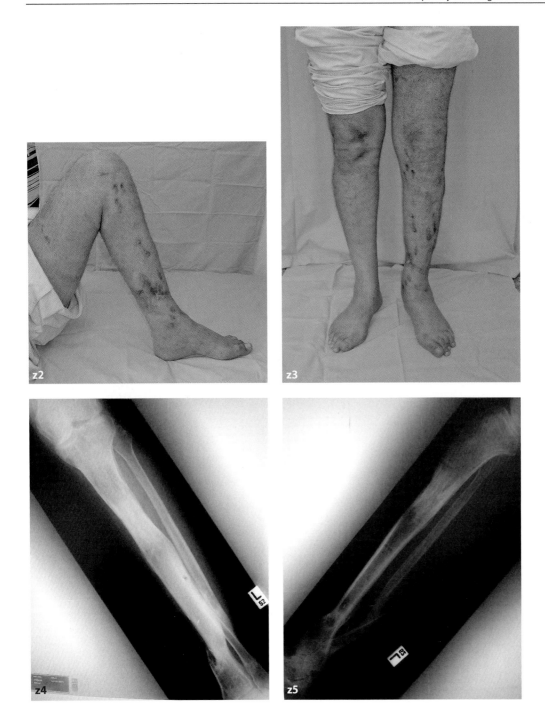

Fig. 3.4.3.2a–z5. *(continued)* **z2–z5** Clinical and radiological photos at follow-up 6 months after removal of the Ilizarov frame. Radiological photos demonstrate bone consolidation of the distal tibial fracture, with solid bone regeneration after completing a 12-cm proximal tibial elongation

Rehabilitation

4

An extensive rehabilitation protocol is the key factor in the postoperative period, especially after peri-articular reconstructions. The rehabilitation arrangements must be started as early as possible and cannot be postponed until the later stages of treatment. Physical therapy should be instituted: muscle strengthening exercises, active and passive mobilization of the injured joints and the joints above and below the injury zone, continuous passive motion machines, electric stimulation, hydrotherapy, and functional use of the injured limbs, as much as possible [102]. Functional mobilization of the hand and fingers, even in more proximally placed injuries of the upper limb, is mandatory. The physiotherapist and occupational therapist have a vital role in encouraging and supervising the earliest possible active and passive movements, and functional recovery. Stable primary fixation of the fracture allows early mobilization of patients, especially those suffering from poly-trauma, avoiding the necessity of prolonged bedrest and its negative consequences. Moreover, it allows the start of mobilization of the non-fixed joints of the injured limb almost immediately (from the first postoperative day).

4.1 Active and Passive Joint Mobilization in External Frames for Treatment of Peri-Articular Injuries

The stability level of the bone fragments must be sufficient to an extent that allows early mobilization and functional loading of the severely injured limb to avoid articular post-traumatic and post-fixation rigidity. Modern basic scientific investigations have shown that early controlled activity promotes healing of injured bones, tendons, ligaments, and skeletal muscles [15]. Thus, the provision of early motions in severely injured joints is a necessary contributing factor in their functional restoration. Active mobilization of the injured limb should commence as soon as the stability of the soft-tissue cover is ensured, including stability of vascular and microvascular anastomoses as well as early healing of the skin grafts [110].

The unilateral external fixator, providing one-sided bone fixation, cannot ensure sufficient fracture stabilization, since it cannot eliminate angulation and rotation forces during functional loading, resulting in loosening of the Schanz screws, pin tract infection, and even loss of fracture alignment. The circular Ilizarov fixator achieves three-dimensional fracture stability, while allowing controlled axial micromotion favorable for bone healing. According to Atesalp et al. [2], the success of the Ilizarov fixator depends on "early function", allowing early joint movement in the treatment of intra-articular fractures. The external fixation method combined with stable fixation of the bone fragments, even in cases of multi-comminuted fractures with minimal surgical traumatization to the soft tissues, provides the conditions necessary for early mobilization. Moreover, accurately placed hinges allow early controlled motion, excluding pathological movements, even in unstable joints. Thus, fracture consolidation and functional rehabilitation are combined. This positively influences the osteoreparation and osteogenesis processes, improves blood circulation, and avoids stiffness.

Usually, active and passive motion must be initiated on the day following surgery. A continuous passive motions machine (CPM) may also be employed. Passive and active exercise of the adjacent joints should be performed each day. After successful coverage of the wounds, and if there are no other medical conditions that require further hospitalization, the patient can continue his or her treatment on an outpatient basic with daily physiotherapeutic treatment and an additional exercise program at home. Remember that prevention of contractures is much simpler than prolonged and not always successful treatment of established contractures (Fig. 4.1.1).

It is necessary to realize that not only flexion-extension motions but also pronation-supination movements are required in the treatment of peri-articular elbow fractures and in the fixation of fractures of the forearm bones in external fixation devices (Fig. 4.1.2).

Separate independent fixation of the humeral, ulnar, and radial bones in hybrid fixation frames achieves these motions even in patients with severe high-energy injuries (Fig. 4.1.3).

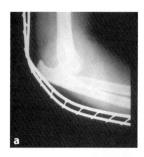
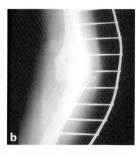
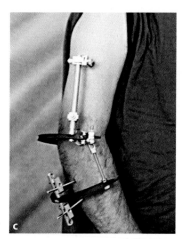
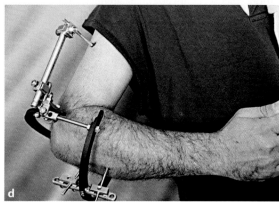
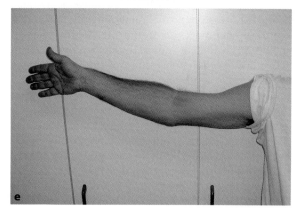
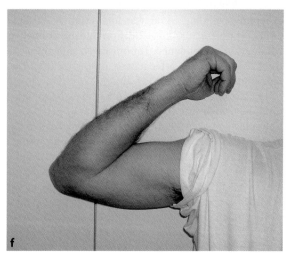

Fig. 4.1.1a–f. A 34-year-old male with elbow joint dislocation due to road traffic accident. The highly unstable elbow joint and secondary displacement was diagnosed on control radiographic examination after closed reduction under general anesthesia and plaster casting. **a,b** Initial radiograph of the right elbow joint demonstrates postero-lateral dislocation of the forearm. **c,d** After repeated reduction of the dislocation, the upper limb is fixed by hinged hybrid external fixation frame. Mobilization of the elbow joint was started immediately after mounting the external frame and continued during the 6-week period of external fixation. **e,f** Clinical appearance after removal of the external fixator

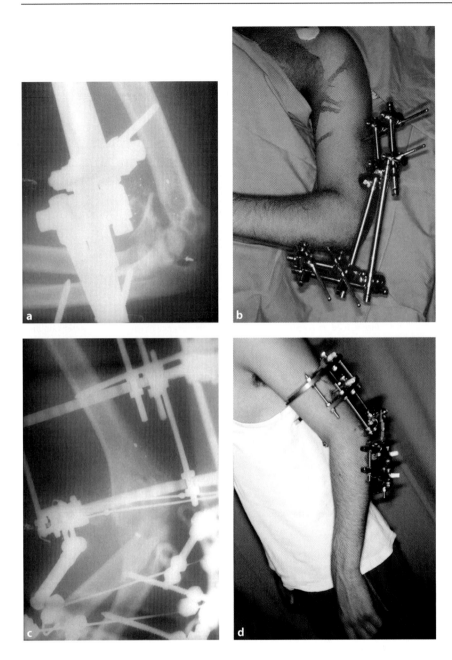

Fig. 4.1.2a–g. A 19-year-old male with open comminuted distal humeral fracture secondary to gunshot. **a,b** Primary debridement and stabilization of the fracture with a unilateral external fixation frame with temporary elbow bridging (radiological and clinical appearance). **c** Closed reduction of the fracture and conversion of unilateral tubular fixator to Ilizarov circular frame performed 5 days later. **d** Clinical appearance of early flexion-extension and pronation-supination movements during fixation in the hinged external fixation frame. **e–g** *see next page*

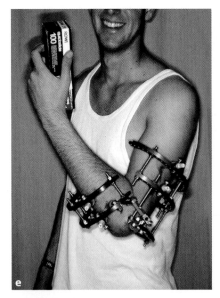

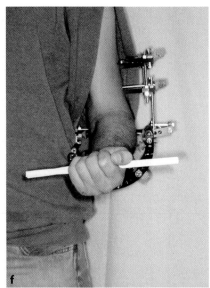

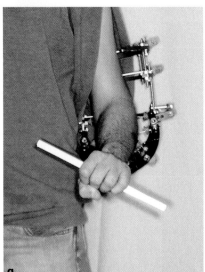

Fig. 4.1.2a–g. *(continued)* **e–g** Clinical appearance of early flexion-extension and pronation-supination movements during fixation in the hinged external fixation frame

Fig. 4.1.3 Clinical appearance of modular isolated external fixation of the humeral, ulnar and radial bones

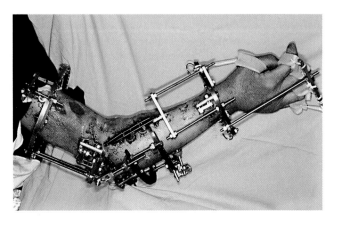

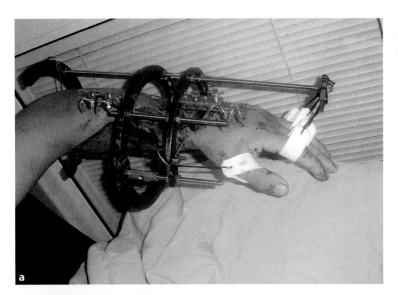

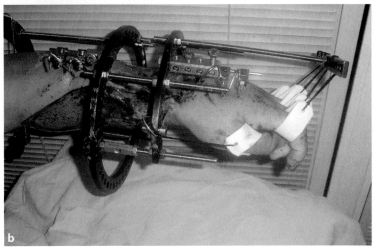

Fig. 4.1.4a,b. Elastic dynamic support to the fingers during external fixation period in treating a severe forearm fracture

Emphasis is placed on preventing finger deformities during the fixation or elongation period. Elastic dynamic finger splints can be useful tools this purpose (Fig. 4.1.4).

The stability of fixation in hybrid/circular Ilizarov frames is sufficient not only for performing active and passive mobilization and physiotherapeutic treatment, but also for holding and using crutches during walking in patients with severe concomitant lower limb injuries (Fig. 4.1.5).

4.2 Weight-Bearing During Stabilization in External Fixation Frame

The Ilizarov circular fixation frame provides effective stabilization even in patients suffering from completely unstable fractures with poor bone apposition or bone loss [64]. Weight-bearing, as tolerated, should be initiated with the help of crutches in patients suffering from severe lower limb injuries during the early postoperative period, according to the wound and soft-tissue condition. There is now evidence that controlled loading of a healing fracture stimulates callus formation and remodeling, and accelerates restoration of bone strength [15, 62]. If there is significant edema, the limb should be kept elevated temporarily. We use a special foot splint, fixed to the frame using elastic straps, to maintain the foot in the plantigrade position. This attachment may also be used for active resisted ankle plantar flexion. Emphasis is placed on keeping the toes in an extended position, preventing claw deformities resulting from post-traumatic muscle imbalance or contracture during bone distraction procedures. A nighttime leg position device is recommended for this purpose for patients with soft-tissue damage to the legs. This device is man-

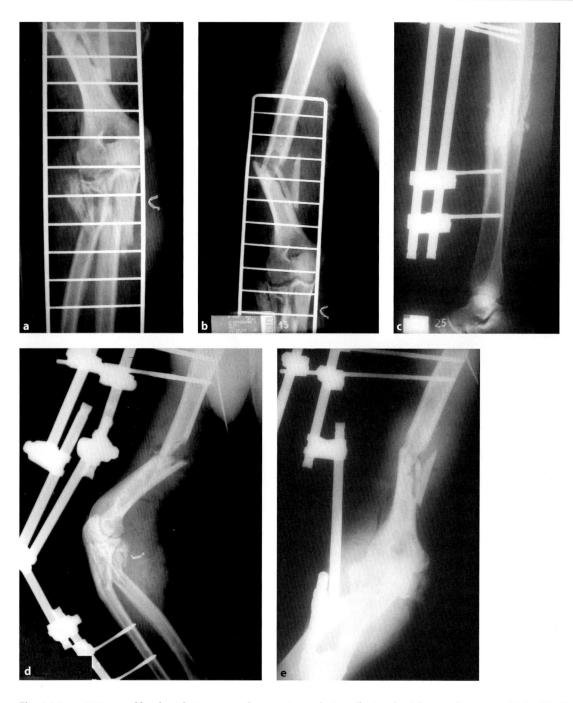

Fig. 4.1.5a–r. A 22-year-old male with injury secondary to mine explosion affecting the right arm, forearm, and right tibia. Emergency treatment was performed, including debridement of open fractures to the limbs and primary stabilization using unilateral external fixation frames. **a,b** Radiographs of right upper limb at time of injury. Comminuted fractures of proximal ulnar, radial, and distal humeral bones. Radiological appearance of multiple foreign bodies in the soft tissue. **c** Radiological appearance of external fixation of the tibial fracture using unilateral frame. **d,e** Radiological and clinical appearance of temporary elbow bridging using unilateral tubular frame. **f–r** *see next page*

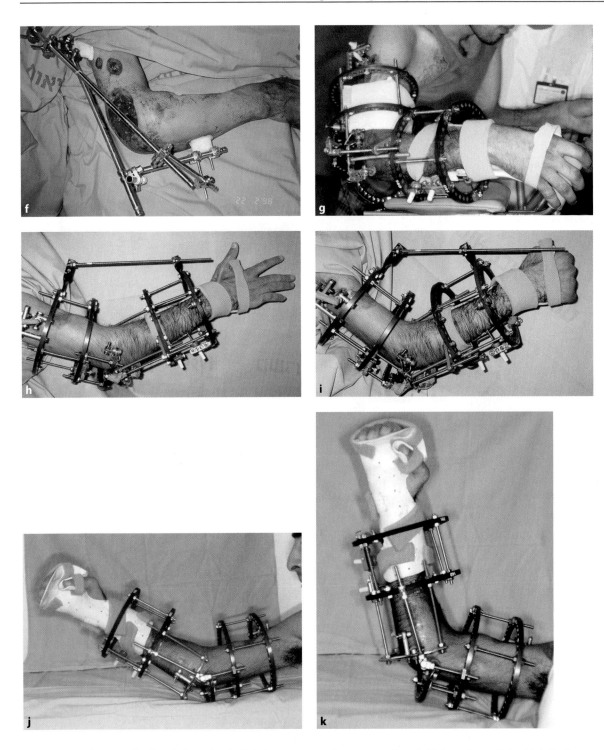

Fig. 4.1.5a–r. *(continued)* **e,f** Radiological and clinical appearance of temporary elbow bridging using unilateral tubular frame. **g** Five days later, the unilateral frame on the upper limb is converted to the Ilizarov hinged frame. **h,i** Temporary absence of active elbow movement due to severe soft-tissue trauma. Clinical appearance of passive mobilization of the elbow joint using additional threaded rod for assisted extension (12 h during daytime) and flexion (12 h during nighttime). **j,k** Three weeks later, active mobilization was started following progress of the soft-tissue condition. **l–r** *see next pages*

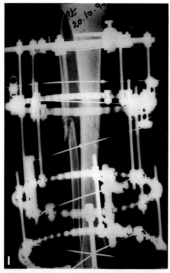

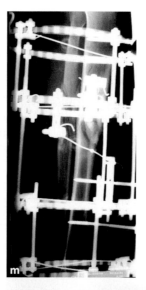

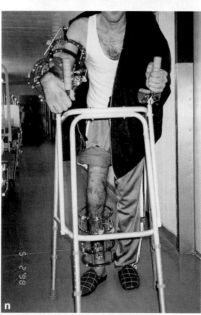

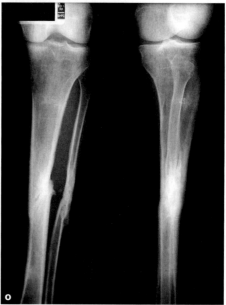

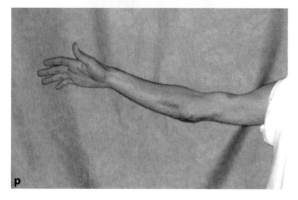

Fig. 4.1.5a–r. *(continued)* **l,m** On the 5th day post-trauma, the tubular external fixator on the tibia was converted to the circular fixation frame (simultaneously with upper limb). **n** Clinical photo demonstrates walking with full weight-bearing to both lower limbs helped by crutching and fixed in the Ilizarov device to the right upper limb. **o** Radiograph of the tibia at follow-up after 12 months. Excellent radiological result has been achieved. **p** Clinical and radiological photos of the upper limb at follow-up after 12 months. **q,r** *see next page*

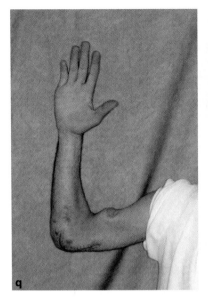
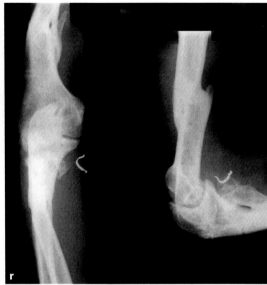

Fig. 4.1.5a–r. *(continued)* **q,r** Clinical and radiological photos of the upper limb at follow-up after 12 months

datory in patients with lower limb lengthening during the period of distraction (Fig. 4.2.1).

In the treatment of patients with lower limb fractures stabilized in external fixation frames, excluding intra-articular ankle fractures and fractures of the foot bones, axial weight-bearing loading to the foot can be allowed using shoes suitable for the patient during standing and walking. This leaves the ankle joint free for active function during walking. Care must be taken to prevent equinus contracture of the ankle and clawing of the toes (Fig. 4.2.2).

In the treatment of patients with more distal fractures, in whom rigid fixation of the foot in the external fixation frame is required, it is possible in some cases to allow partial weight-bearing on the foot using a thick elastic sole tied to the foot with an external fixation ring (Fig. 4.2.3).

When any loading on the foot is undesirable (foot fractures, not stably fixed, or multi-comminuted fractures around the ankle joint, or significant shortening of the injured limb) weight-bearing during walking is performed via a metallic bar attached to the rings and remote from the foot. Even when weight-bearing is not possible, early range of motion exercises of the foot and ankle joint may prevent post-traumatic stiffness, edema, and reflex sympathetic dystrophy (Fig. 4.2.4).

The desired level of stability to be provided optimally by the external fixation frame differs during various stages of treatment, and is inversely proportional to the rigidity of the bone callus. According to Catagni [19], the Ilizarov device provides a certain amount of needed elasticity but does not compromise the overall stability

of the bone-fixator complex; the Ilizarov frame provides a proper balance between elasticity and stability. After healing of the soft-tissue wound, patients can live at home, and long-term treatments, including gradual realignment of the bone fragments or elongation procedures, are performed in an outpatient setting.

The risk of re-fracture associated with premature removal of the external fixation frame should be considered, especially in patients with significant stiffness in the adjacent joints. In this case, the frame can by remove gradually, using a method of staged withdrawal of one or two fixation elements (thin wires or half-pins) at each control outpatient examination. Thus, a gradual diminishing of the stabilization properties of the external fixation frame leads to increased functional loading on the healing bone during this prolonged process of de-mounting the frame. This can be an important factor in the acceleration of the bone healing process under conditions of minimal external support, the so-called education of the bone regeneration. Another simple method of dynamization allows weight-bearing in the presence of fully loosened threaded rods above the fracture site in the final stage of external fixation, when good callus formation is apparent on the control radiographic examination. Solomin [119] proposed an interesting method regarding "modular transformation of the fixation frame": gradually diminishing the number of fixation elements of the external frame, including thin wires, half-pins, threaded rods, and half-rings.

It must be kept in mind that, in treating patients suffering from high-energy trauma, especially gunshot and blast injuries, bone healing is usually slower

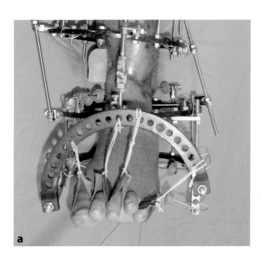

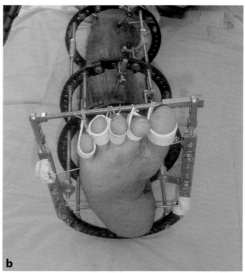

Fig. 4.2.1a,b. Clinical appearance of elastic dynamic support to the toes used during period of bone elongation and external fixation

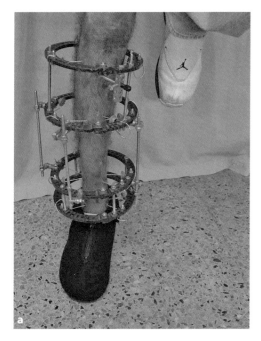

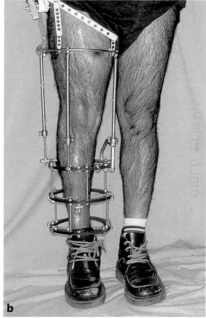

Fig. 4.2.2a–e. Clinical appearance of weight-bearing during external fixation period in Ilizarov circular device using regular shoe

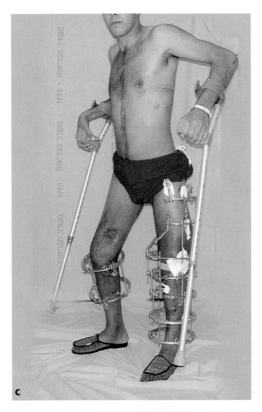

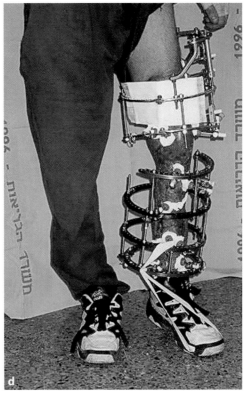

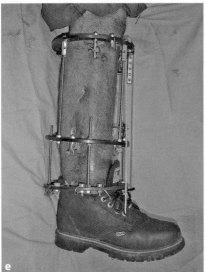

Fig. 4.2.2a–e. *(continued)* Clinical appearance of weight-bearing during external fixation period in Ilizarov circular device using regular shoe

than in low-energy injuries. Thus, the period of external fixation may be very prolonged. It is desirable, in questionable cases, for external fixation of the fracture to be continued, avoiding premature removal of the fixation frame. In performing de-mounting of the external frame, we start the procedure by removing the connecting threaded rods above the fracture site, and not by extracting the thin wires and half-pins. Signs of pathological mobility in the fracture zone demand a return to fastening the rods and continuing the external fixation. After removing the external fixation frames, plaster casts or braces are usually applied to protect the limbs from re-fracture for a few weeks. Weight-bearing loading is continued during this bracing stage.

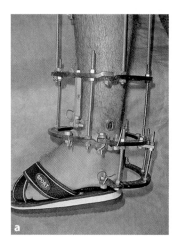

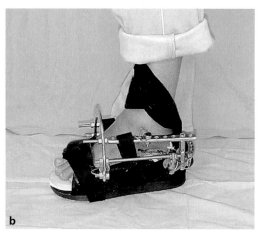

Fig. 4.2.3a,b. Clinical appearance of the high elastic sole tied to the foot ring used for weight-bearing with expansion of the external fixation frame to the foot

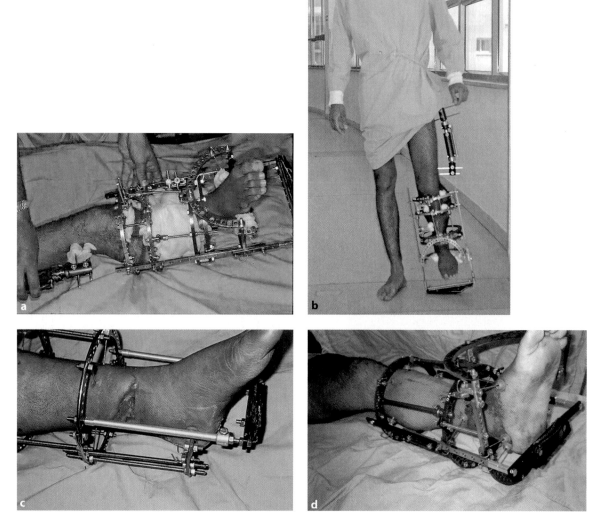

Fig. 4.2.4a–d. Clinical appearance of the metal "horse-shoe" attachment to the frame, used for transfer of weight-bearing loading forces to the more proximally placed rings of the circular fixation frame

Treatment Algorithm for Missile Open Fractures of the Limbs

5

A simple classification system could be a useful working tool in treating complex war injuries to the extremities. However, there is no consensus on a universal work classification, because these patients are a highly heterogeneous group, making comparisons and conclusions difficult. Various classifications have been elaborated over time, but a validated and universally accepted classification system has yet to be developed. Existing trauma classification systems do not address the distinctive nature, complexity, and severity of these injuries [42]. According to Keating et al. [61], due to the large number of factors which determine the severity and outcome of these injuries, none of the existing schemes is entirely satisfactory. Several scoring systems have been devised to assist in predicting successful limb salvage, but these scores do not work well in clinical practice, especially in patients with high-energy war injuries, where a significant number of the cases manifest an unusual situation. The Gustilo–Anderson classification system [44, 45] is commonly used for evaluating open fractures and deciding on appropriate treatment [48]. The most important factor in this system is the size of the wound, but this parameter does not always reflect the degree and extent of soft-tissue damage in the depth of the wound, which finally determine the prognosis of treatment. Severe and widespread soft tissue destruction is very frequent in war injuries and often does not correspond to the entry wound size [87]. Misclassification of an open fracture can occur, especially in a patient with a relatively small skin wound, and the extent and severity of the injury should be assessed only during surgery, after wound exploration and debridement, and not at presentation in the emergency department [146]. In patients suffering from high-energy injuries, especially crush and blast injuries, the condition of the injured limbs can be assessed only during repeated debridement procedures.

Ganocy and Lindsey [39] proposed a classification system for civilian intra-articular gunshot wounds that included three key factors – bullet location, contamination, and fracture – with a treatment algorithm based on three important variables and on three possible levels of severity. Gugala and Lindsey [42] proposed a more complex classification system of gunshot injuries in civilians – including parameters of energy, vital structure damage, wound characteristic, type of fracture, grade of contamination – which determines the clinical parameters for surgical treatment. Shepherd and colleagues [114] evaluated the reliability of the AO/Orthopaedic Trauma Association classification system for gunshot femoral shaft fractures and concluded that they cannot be classified reliably with this classification system. The Mangled Extremity Severity Score (MESS) classification is not precise enough to allow a decision regarding amputation to be made at initial surgery [37]. According to Durham et al. [31], the Mangled Extremity Scoring Index (MESI), MESS, the Predictive Salvage Index (PSI), and the Limb Salvage Index (LSI) as predictors of amputation and functional outcome in severe blunt extremity trauma were unable to predict functional outcome.

The Red Cross Classification of War Wounds was proposed for firearm injuries and is preferred by some authors [10, 11, 21, 23] for evaluating patients suffering from war injuries. Its E.X.C.F.V.M. Scoring System is also based upon features of the wound but not upon weaponry. These classifications do not reflect the quantity of energy absorbed by the soft and hard tissues. Moreover, the presence of numerous parameters in the classification system leads to significant complications in its use. Some severe specific conditions, especially those caused by land mines, are insufficiently defined or unmarked in international classifications [46].

A detailed history of the mechanism of injury, early clinical and radiographic signs and symptoms can be of great help in gaining a clear understanding of the general and local condition and the choice of the correct management tactic for patients suffering from high-energy war injuries [142]. Extensive destruction due to wounding with projectiles of high kinetic energy (initial velocity), and especially in cases of blast injuries, is the frequent presentation in war injuries. Not only high-velocity bullets but also low-velocity weapons can result in high-energy tissue damage, depending on the distance, bullet caliber, and wounding potential. Massive bone comminution producing secondary missiles, such as bony fragments, may produce massive tissue damage [42]. According to Bartlett et al. [5], most low-velocity gunshot wounds can be safely treated non-operatively with local wound care and outpatient management. Formal surgical debridement is not always necessary if the accompanying soft-tissue damage is not extensive [133]. The guidelines for treating high-energy war injuries have not been standardized.

Patients suffering from low-energy trauma may present with extremely variable injuries [39]. This diversity is even more apparent in cases of high-energy war trauma, especially due to blast. Taking into account this diversity, it follows that a classification of war combat injuries can be unwieldy and intricate, if it tries to take into consideration all the possible separate details of the trauma. We contend that a firearm injuries classification must be based in the first place on the quantity of the energy absorbed by the tissues. The latter determines the severity and extent of the tissue damage and the prognosis. The line between injuries inflicted by low-velocity and high-velocity weapons is not always clear cut. When in doubt, the injury is assessed as severe and given the appropriate treatment.

Based on our experience in treating patients with high-velocity fractures, we propose a treatment protocol according to the amount of energy absorbed by the tissues. This classification system also has practical implications as it can assist in the selection of proper treatment. The soft-tissue trauma is the most important component of the high-energy injury, dictating the initial and sometimes definitive management of the traumatized extremity [102]. High-energy injuries result in increased comminuting and less predictable fracture patterns. High-energy fractures are frequently associated with significant injury to the soft-tissue envelope that demands special consideration and which may affect treatment options. In patients with high-energy injuries, infection is promoted by bacterial contamination and colonization of the wound, the presence of dead space with devitalized tissues, foreign material, and the compromised host response resulting from poor vascularity and soft-tissue damage [146]. Thus, high-energy injuries usually have a combination of significant tissue destruction with severe reconstruction dilemmas, difficult operative procedures, challenging postoperative rehabilitation and uncertain outcomes [144].

Soft tissues assume a most critical role in the accurate prognosis and selection of adequate treatment approaches for the management of patients with high-velocity and gunshot wounds. According to a study by MacKenzie et al. [90] to evaluate factors influencing the decision to perform amputation of lower limbs after high-energy trauma, the degree of bone loss was not a significant factor. Severity of soft-tissue damage, including absence of plantar sensation, was the most important consideration.

Table 1 Primary treatment algorithm for open missile fractures of the limbs

	Type	Primary treatment
Low-velocity gunshot injuries	1. Simple fractures	Debridement. Internal or external fixation
	2. Vascular compromised fractures	Debridement. Internal or external fixation. Vascular repair
High-energy injuries	1. High-velocity gunshot wounds + close-range low-velocity gunshot wounds	
	a. Shaft fractures	Debridement. External fixation
	b. Intra-articular fractures	Debridement. Temporary trans-articular external fixation. Early exchange of joint bridging to fracture fixation
	c. Open fractures with severe soft-tissue loss	Debridement. External fixation. Early soft-tissue coverage (acute shortening with/without angulation or flaps)
	d. Vascular compromised fractures	Debridement. External fixation. Vascular repair
	2. Explosion injuries	
	a. Shrapnel wounds	Debridement. External fixation. Early soft-tissue coverage (acute shortening with/without angulation or flaps)
	b. Shrapnel wounds + Crush	Debridement. External fixation. Early soft-tissue coverage (acute shortening with/without angulation or flaps)
	c. Post-traumatic segmental absence of limb	Completion of the amputation with open stump

Conclusions

High-energy limb injuries, especially in patients suffering from war trauma, often result in severe and extensive tissue loss and tissue devascularization, creating a high rate of complications, thereby increasing overall morbidity [45, 49, 80, 137]. In the management of massive limb wounds, the appropriate treatment must take into consideration the nature of the injury, the surgical insult and technique, and a variety of patient factors, but the nature of the injury is the most important factor when a management decision is made [101]. According to Celikoz et al. [20], early, aggressive, and serial debridement of osseous and soft tissue, restoration of bone and soft-tissue defects, intensive rehabilitation, and patient education were the key points in the management of high-velocity, high-energy injuries to limbs. Before concentrating our attention on the extremity injury, any potential life-threatening problems must be assessed and managed. In our experience, a staged protocol of external fixation, including primary temporary unilateral tubular stabilization, followed by definitive circular or hybrid fixation in a customized frame is an effective method for the management of patients suffering from severe damage to the bone and soft tissues due to high-energy war injuries. Careful attention to soft-tissue integrity begins at the first examination of the injury and dictates timing, incisions, and eventual mode of surgical treatment [7]. High-energy and contaminated wounds require immediate and aggressive irrigation and debridement with thorough excision of necrotic tissues and fascial decompression. The greatest challenge, and the greatest importance for the orthopedic surgeon is achieving as perfect as possible debridement of the wound. Ineffective fracture stabilization causes additional soft-tissue damage and morbidity, pain, and severe nursing problems during treatment. Contrarily, early skeletal stabilization improves the recovery of overlying soft tissues and facilitates nursing care.

Historically, attempts at open reduction and internal fixation of high-energy fractures have been associated with high rates of wound complication [33]. Nowadays, rates of infection after open reduction and internal fixation for the treatment of open fractures are significantly reduced due to improved surgical skills in accordance with biological principles of less invasive techniques of fracture reduction and fixation – principles of "biological fixation." Moreover, the use of external fixation frames in the initial phase of the treatment of patients with severe high-energy injuries provides improved results of treatment. The stable external fracture fixation allows early mobilization of the patients which facilitates nursing care and avoids many complications in the poly-traumatized patients. Application of this method does not aggravate the patient's general condition. External fixation frames are especially favored in the treatment of patients with extensive soft-tissue damage because stabilization can be achieved easily, further soft-tissue dissection is not needed, and soft-tissue care is facilitated; versatile modern external fixation frames may be deployed in almost any location and fracture pattern. Benefits of the use of temporary external fixation until the soft-tissue envelope has sufficiently healed, followed by definitive internal fixation, have been demonstrated by several authors in treating complex distal femoral and proximal and distal tibial fractures. The use of two-stage reconstruction for the treatment of complex limb fractures has been successful in decreasing complication rates [9, 47, 134]. The two stages involve: (1) stabilization of the injured limb with a bridging external fixator to allow the soft tissues to improve and recover, and (2) definitive reconstruction and fixation of complex fractures.

The staged treatment protocol with conversion from primary tubular external fixation to internal fixation has been well described and accepted for the management of patients suffering from multiple trauma or from open low-energy fractures, and also in the treatment of some patients after open high-energy trauma where there is no severe tissue loss and good coverage of the fracture site can be achieved. The primary benefit of such a protocol is the reduction in soft-tissue complications as compared with immediate open surgery [109]. Haidukewych [47] wrote that the method of temporary external fixation in patients with severe limb trauma can be summarized by the word "prepare": preparing the severely injured patient, preparing the injured extremity, and preparing the surgeon for the definitive complex reconstructive procedure. Currently, this staged protocol of treatment of temporary external fixation, followed by formal open reduction and internal fixation (including limited open reduction and minimal internal fixation, combined with additional external stabilization) is an accepted method for dealing with this type of injury [1, 47, 140].

When the tissues have absorbed a high quantity of energy, especially when adequate soft-tissue coverage is lacking, the probability of deep infection is increased. Post-traumatic osteomyelitis, demanding long-term treatment including multiple complex operative procedures, is the result of these conditions (Fig. 6.1).

Localization of the massive internal fixation device in the depth of the wound can aggravate disturbances in the local tissue blood supply and cause a septic process along the implanted foreign body (Fig. 6.2).

In contrast, the staged external fixation protocol provides conditions for a minimally traumatic surgical reconstruction, providing a safe method with respect to the soft-tissue envelope [84]. Improved blood supply to the fracture site may translate into improved rates of union, decreased rates of bone grafting, decreased incidents of non-union, re-fractures and deep infection. On the day of admission, the fractured bones are re-aligned and stabilized with an AO/ASIF tubular external fixator, followed by immediate extensive soft-tissue debridement and cleansing. The next stage of treatment is conversion of the unilateral fixation frame to the circular Ilizarov frame. The low morbidity associated with the Ilizarov method suits it to the management of complex fractures when extensive dissection and internal fixation are contraindicated due to comminution at the fracture site and extensive damage to the soft tissue [27]. The Ilizarov method is not only a method of surgical fracture fixation; it also provides a unique continuous, guided, active influence on tissue healing and reshaping, with functional restoration under the complex conditions of high-energy injury with extensive tissue damage and loss.

The versatility of the current external fixation systems provides the best means for fast and safe stabilization of severe open fractures, especially in using unilateral tubular systems. In contrast, circular external fixation is the most technically demanding fixation method, requiring a complete mastery of surgical anatomy and basic technical principles. Optimal treatment of bone fractures should include: (1) anatomical reduction, (2) stable fixation, and (3) early mobilization (weight-bearing in lower limb injuries). Modern modular circular/hybrid external fixation frames can satisfy all these demands based principally on percutaneous surgery. This second-stage reconstructive procedure must be performed electively by a team of experienced trauma orthopedic surgeons. Moreover, successful application of the method requires careful follow-up of patients throughout the entire healing process.

Staged external fixation is a valuable treatment strategy for providing stability to extremities with high-energy and war injuries. This treatment strategy is a complex of logically interrelated measures for the preservation and functional restoration of severely injured limbs with extensive tissue loss (both bone and soft tissue), using the method of modular circular/hybrid external fixation. The method allows restoration of the shape and function of the injured limb without a need for massive implanted devices, and avoids traumatic methods of tissue transfer in many patients. In unstable poly-traumatized patients and those with combined soft tissue injuries (i.e., degloving, burns), stabilization of the fracture by external fixation allows early mobilization of the patient, and facilitates nursing care.

Considerable variation in the configuration and extent of tissue damage in patients suffering from high-energy trauma dictates that prescriptive management based on an established protocol is not possible: a flexible and individualized approach to treatment is required [61].

The unique abilities of the Ilizarov method in the restoration of extensive bone defects without needing massive bone grafting allow the orthopedic surgeon more freedom during the performance of the most vital part of the treatment in the high-energy trauma patient – namely, the primary surgical debridement procedure. Primary stabilization of the injured limb in a position of temporary malposition (shortening, angulation, rotation) will reduce the size of the skin and soft-tissue defect and may avoid the need for traumatic and technically demanding local, distant and free soft-tissue flaps. Definitive bone reconstruction can be delayed until soft-tissue problems are solved. Later, after successful soft-tissue coverage and healing, bone restoration can be performed gradually in a minimally traumatic manner. Patient compliance is an absolute requirement for the successful result of such a complex, prolonged treatment process of serial planned and unplanned surgical interventions (named the "preamputation limb salvage option" by Rozbruch et al. [111]).

In summary, a staged protocol of external fixation, including primary temporary unilateral tubular stabilization followed by definitive circular (hybrid) fixation by customized frame, is an effective tool in the treatment of patients with severe compound damage to the bone and soft tissues with poor local biological conditions due to high-energy trauma, including war injuries [84]. This staged treatment protocol is an effective method of management in mass casualty conditions, such as terror attacks, war, industrial accidents, train and nature cataclysms. Our clinical experience emphasizes the versatility of this approach and the relatively low morbidity associated with this minimally invasive method.

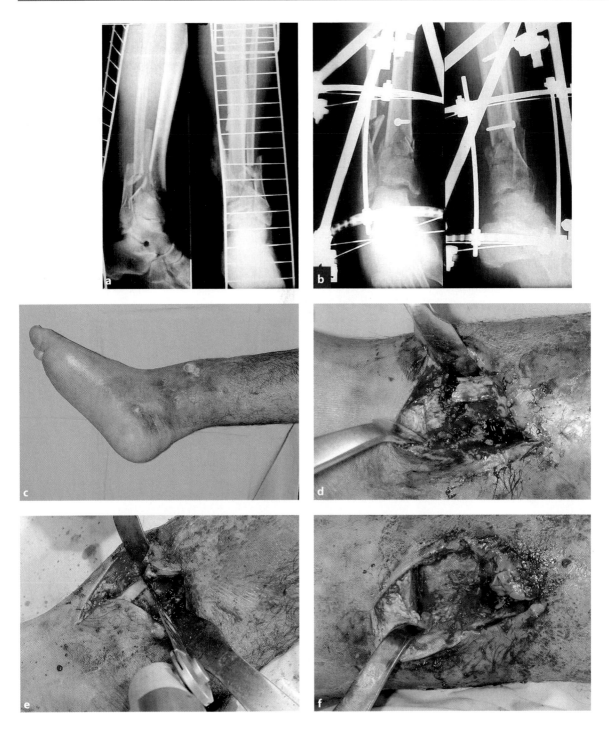

Fig. 6.1a–m. A 36-year old male with open Gustilo type IIIA right distal tibial fracture due to work accident. **a** Radiograph at admission demonstrates displaced comminuted fractures of the distal third of right tibial and fibular bones. **b** Primary emergency care was carried out. Debridement of soft tissues, and stabilizing the tibial fracture using minimal internal fixation by inter-fragmentary screw combined with a hybrid external fixation frame were performed. Postoperative radiological appearance demonstrates anatomical reduction of the tibial bone. **c** Postoperative period was complicated by infected wound, post-traumatic osteomyelitis and non-union. Deformation of the leg with pathological movements in the fracture site and suppurating wound after removal of the external fixation frame were diagnosed (clinical picture). **d–f** Debridement of septic focus, sequestrectomy with segmental resection of the infected bone, was performed. Total bone defect is 6 cm (clinical photos). **g–m** *see next page*

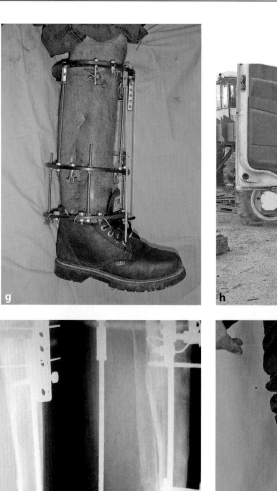

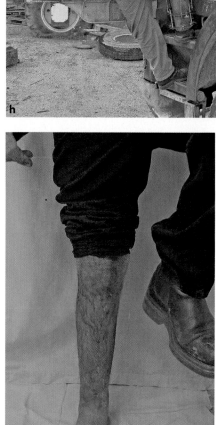

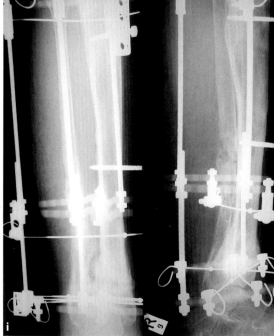

Fig. 6.1a–m. *(continued)* **g** The leg was stabilized using an Ilizarov frame. Three weeks later, proximal tibial corticotomy for leg length restoration was performed (postoperative clinical photo). **h** Post-resection distal tibial defect was completely restored by a technique of controlled gradual distraction in the zone of the proximal tibial corticotomy. During the treatment period, the patient was fully ambulatory, living at home and working as a locksmith (clinical photo at work during period of external fixation in the Ilizarov frame). **i** Radiograph after 9 months of Ilizarov external fixation demonstrates consolidation at the distal tibial fracture and good bone regeneration at the site of proximal tibial elongation corticotomy. **j** Total time of external tibial fixation: 13 months. Clinical photos at follow-up 2 years after removal of the Ilizarov frame, showing complete restoration of the right lower limb length and shape. No length discrepancy resulted. Near to full range of ankle movement is preserved. Tibial non-union and infection process are healed. **k–m** *see next page*

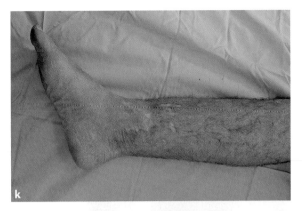

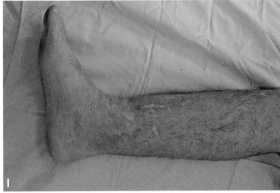

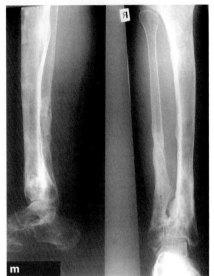

Fig. 6.1a–m. *(continued)* **k,l** Total time of external tibial fixation: 13 months. Clinical photos at follow-up 2 years after removal of the Ilizarov frame, showing complete restoration of the right lower limb length and shape. No length discrepancy resulted. Near to full range of ankle movement is preserved. Tibial nonunion and infection process are healed. **m** Radiological photos at the 2-year follow-up demonstrate complete bone healing of the tibial fracture, solid bone regeneration after completion of 6-cm proximal tibial bone elongation

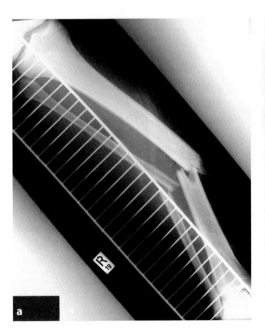

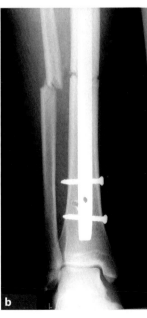

Fig. 6.2a–z. A 19-year-old male suffering from open Gustilo type IIIB right tibial fracture due to fall from the third floor. **a** Radiograph on admission demonstrates displaced midshaft fracture of the right tibial and fibular bones. **b** Primary emergency care was carried out with debridement of the soft tissues, stabilizing the tibial fracture using reamed locked intramedullary nail, and coverage of the fracture site by local rotational fasciocutaneous flap. Radiological appearance after internal fixation demonstrates anatomical reduction of the tibial bone. **c–z** *see next page*

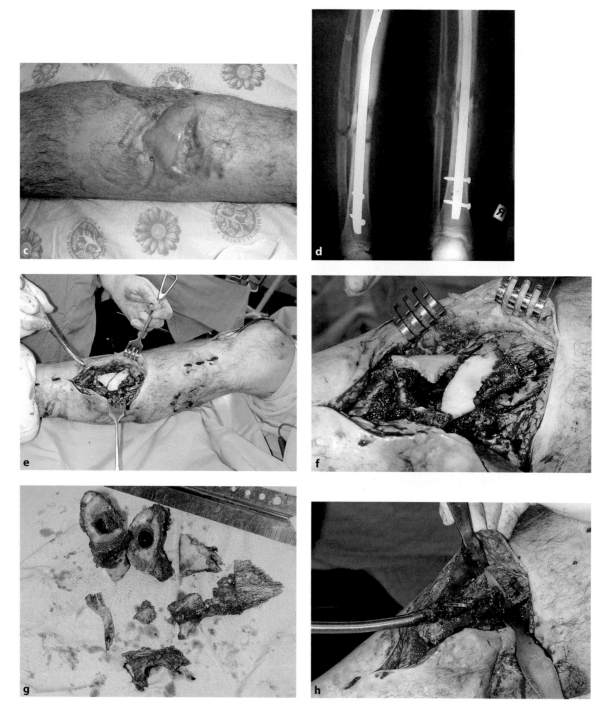

Fig. 6.2a–z. *(continued)* **c** Procedures are complicated by infected wound (clinical photo). **d** Radiological examination 2 months later demonstrates signs of osteomyelitis with sequestration of the tibial bone. **e–g** Debridement of septic focus, sequestrectomy with segmental resection of the infected bone, was performed. **h** Debridement of the medullary canal by drilling and brushing was done. Total bone defect was 7 cm. **i–z** *see next page*

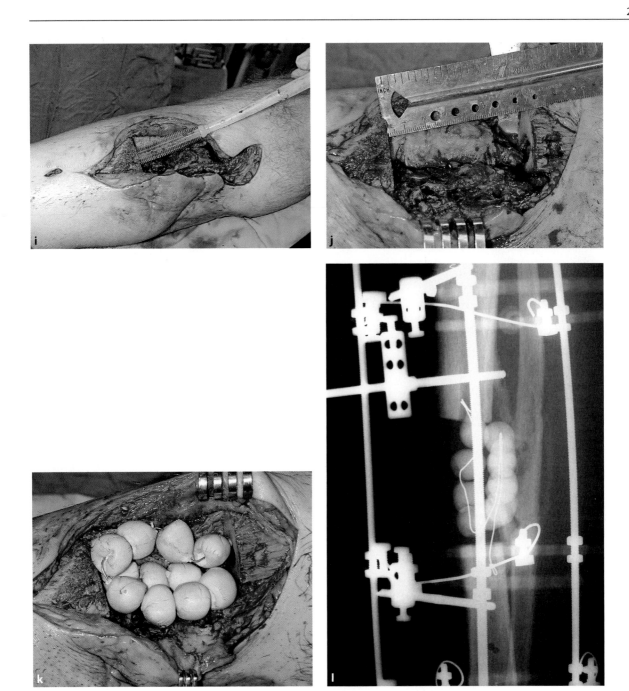

Fig. 6.2a–z. *(continued)* **i,j** Debridement of the medullary canal by drilling and brushing was done. Total bone defect was 7 cm. **k** Antibiotic beads were placed to the site of the tibial bone defect. **l** Stabilization using an Ilizarov frame was performed (postoperative radiological and clinical photos). **m–z** *see next page*

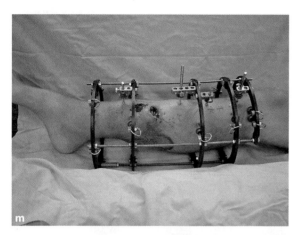

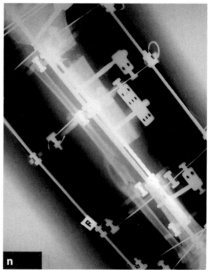

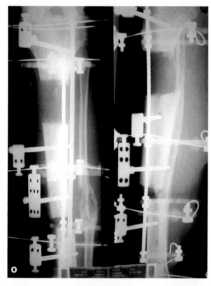

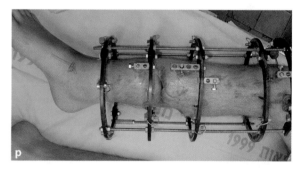

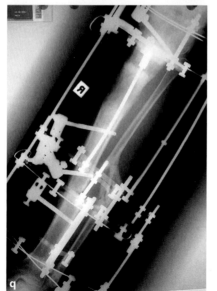

Fig. 6.2a–z. *(continued)* **m** Stabilization using an Ilizarov frame was performed (postoperative radiological and clinical photos). **n** Three weeks later, the antibiotic beads were removed and proximal tibial corticotomy for bone transport was performed. Radiological photo after 2 weeks of bone transport demonstrates gap at the site of tibial corticotomy. **o,p** Skin invagination at the docking site (clinical photo) was observed after 2 months of bone transport (radiological photo). Bone transport was temporarily stopped at this stage, and surgical correction of the invaginated skin was performed. **q** Stoppage of the bone transport resulted in premature bone regenerate consolidation. Repeat proximal tibial corticotomy was needed to allow bone transport continuation (radiological photos demonstrate site of repeated corticotomy). **r–z** *see next page*

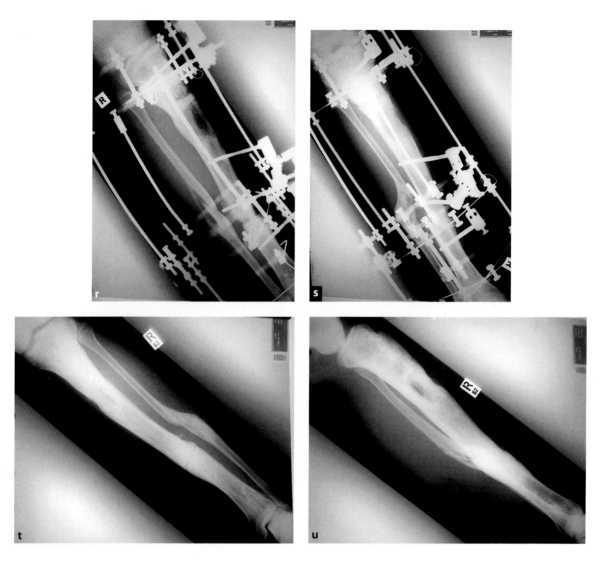

Fig. 6.2a–z. *(continued)* **r** Stoppage of the bone transport resulted in premature bone regenerate consolidation. Repeat proximal tibial corticotomy was needed to allow bone transport continuation (radiological photos demonstrate site of repeated corticotomy). **s** Post-resection tibial defect was completely restored by bone transport technique (X-ray). Total time for external tibial fixation: 15 months. **t,u** Radiological photos at the 2-year follow-up demonstrate complete bone healing of the tibial fracture and solid bone regeneration after completion of 7-cm proximal bone transport **(v–z)**. Clinical photos at follow-up 2 years after removal of the Ilizarov frame, showing complete restoration of the right lower limb length and shape. No length discrepancy resulted. Complete range of knee and ankle movements are preserved. Non-union and infection process are healed. **v–z** *see next page*

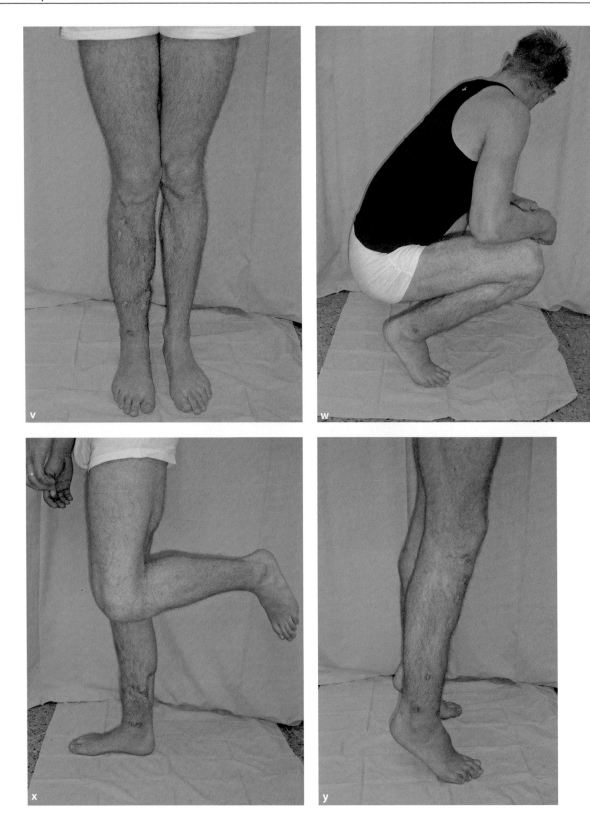

Fig. 6.2a–z. *(continued)* **v–y** Radiological photos at the 2-year follow-up demonstrate complete bone healing of the tibial fracture and solid bone regeneration after completion of 7-cm proximal bone transport **(v–z)**. Clinical photos at follow-up 2 years after removal of the Ilizarov frame, showing complete restoration of the right lower limb length and shape. No length discrepancy resulted. Complete range of knee and ankle movements are preserved. Non-union and infection process are healed. **z** *see next page*

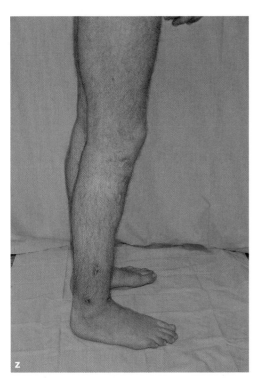

Fig. 6.2a–z. *(continued)* **z** Radiological photos at the 2-year follow-up demonstrate complete bone healing of the tibial fracture and solid bone regeneration after completion of 7-cm proximal bone transport (**v–z**). Clinical photos at follow-up 2 years after removal of the Ilizarov frame, showing complete restoration of the right lower limb length and shape. No length discrepancy resulted. Complete range of knee and ankle movements are preserved. Non-union and infection process are healed

References

1. Anglen JO, Aleto T (1998) Temporary transarticular external fixation of the knee and ankle. J Orthop Trauma 12:431–434

2. Atesalp AS, Yildiz C, Basboskurt M et al (2002) Treatment of type IIIA open fractures with Ilizarov fixation and delayed primary closure in high-velocity gunshot wounds. Mil Med 167:56–62

3. Barr RJ, Mollan RAB (1989) The orthopaedic consequences of civil disturbance in Northern Ireland. J Bone Joint Surg 71B:739–744

4. Bartlett C (2003) Clinical update: gunshot wound ballistics. Clin Orthop 408:28–57

5. Bartlett C, Helfet D, Hausman M (2000) Ballistic and gunshot wounds: effects on musculoskeletal tissues. J Am Acad Orthop Surg 8:21–36

6. Behrens F, Johnson (1989) Unilateral external fixation. Methods to increase and reduce frame stiffness. Clin Orthop Relat Res 241:48–56

7. Berkson EM, Virkus WW (2006) High-energy tibial plateau fractures. J Am Acad Orthop Surg 14:20–31

8. Bilic R, Kolundzic R, Bicanic G et al (2005) Elbow arthrodesis after war injuries. Mil Med 170:164–166

9. Blachut PA, Meek RN, O'Brien PJ (1990) External fixation and delayed intramedullary nailing of open fractures of the tibial shaft: a sequential protocol. J Bone Joint Surg 72A:729–735

10. Bowyer GW (1995) Afghan war wounded: application of the Red Cross wound classification. J Trauma 38:64–67

11. Bowyer GW, Stewart MP, Ryan JM (1993) Gulf war wounds: application of the Red Cross wound classification. Injury 24:597–600

12. Brettler D, Sedlin ED, Mendes DG (1979) Conservative treatment of low velocity gunshot wounds. Clin Orthop 140:26–31

13. Brien WW, Kushner SH, Brien E et al (1995) The management of gunshot wounds to the femur. Ortho Clin North Am 26:133–138

14. Brusov PG, Shapovalov VM, Artemiev AA et al (1996) Combat injuries to the limbs [in Russian]. Geotar, Moscow, p 130

15. Buckwalter JA, Grodzinsky AJ (1999) Loading of healing bone, fibrous tissue, and muscle: implications for orthopaedic practice. J Am Acad Orthop Surg 7:291–299

16. Busic Z, Lovric Z, Amic E et al (2006) War injuries of the extremities: twelve-year follow-up data. Mil Med 171:55–57

17. Calif E, Stein H, Lerner A (2004) The Ilizarov external fixation frame in compression arthrodesis of large, weight bearing joints. Acta Orthopaed Belg 70 (1):51–56

18. Canocy K II, Lindsey RW (1997) The management of civilian intra-articular gunshot wounds: treatment considerations and proposal of a classification system. Injury 29 [Suppl 1]:SA1–SA6

19. Catagni M (1998) Treatment of fractures, nonunions, and bone loss of the tibia with the Ilizarov method. Medical-plastic, Milan, Italy

20. Celikoz B, Sengezer M, Isik S et al (2005) Subacute reconstruction of lower leg and foot defects due to high velocity-high energy injuries caused by gunshots, missiles, and land mines. Microsurgery 25:3–14

21. Cernak I, Savic J, Zunic G et al (1999) Recognizing, scoring, and predicting blast injuries. World J Surg 23:44–53

22. Coupland RM (1989) Technical aspects of war wounds excision. Br J Surg 76:663–667

23. Coupland RM (1992) The Red Cross classification of war wounds: the E.X.C.F.V.M scoring system. World J Surg 16:910–917

24. Davila S, Mikulic D, Davila NJ et al (2005) Treatment of war injuries of the shoulder with external fixators. Mil Med 170:414–417

25. DeFranzo AJ, Argenta LC, Marks MW et al (2001) The use of vacuum assisted closure therapy for the treatment of lower extremity wounds with exposed bone. Plast Reconstr Surg 108:1184–1191

26. Deitch EA, Grimes WR (1984) Experience with 112 shotgun wounds of the extremities. J Trauma 24:600–612

27. Dendrinos GK, Kontos S, Katsenis D et al (1996) Treatment of high-energy tibial plateau fractures by the Ilizarov circular fixator. J Bone Joint Surg 78B:710–717

28. Dillman R, Crumb C, Lidsky M (1979) Lead poisoning from a gunshot wound. Report of a case and review of the literature. Am J Med 66:509–514

29. Draeger RW, Dahners LE (2006) Traumatic wound debridement. A comparison of irrigation methods. J Orthop Trauma 20:83–88

30. Duman H, Sengezer M, Celikoz B et al (2001) Lower extremity salvage using a free flap associated with the Ilizarov method in patients with massive combat injuries. Ann Plast Surg 46:108–112

31. Durham RM, Mistry BM, Mazuski JE et al (1996) Outcome and utility of scoring systems in the management of the mangled extremity. Am J Surg 172:569–573

32. Efimenko NA, Shapovalov VM, Dulaev AK et al (2003) Characteristic of combat trauma and treatment of gunshot fractures of long bones of the limbs [in Russian]. Voen Med Zh 324:4–12, 80

33. Egol KA, Tejwani NC, Capla EL et al (2005) Staged management of high-energy proximal tibia fractures (OTA types 41) The results of the prospective standardized protocol. J Orthop Trauma 19:448–455

34. Fackler ML (1995) Wound ballistics and soft-tissue wound management. Techniques Orthop 10:163–170

35. Fackler ML, Surinchak JS, Malinowski BS et al (1984) Bullet fragmentation a major case of tissue disruption. J Trauma 24:35–39

36. Fackler ML, Bellamy RF, Malinowski JA (1988) The wound profile: illustration of the missile-tissue interaction. J Trauma 28B [Suppl 1]:S21–S29

37. Faris IB, Raptis S, Fitridge R (1997) Arterial injury in the limb from blunt trauma. Aust NZ J Surg 67:25–30

38. Fox CJ, Gillespie DL, O'Donnell SD et al (2005) Contemporary management of wartime vascular trauma. J Vasc Surg 41:638–644

39. Ganocy K, Lindsey RW 2nd (1998) The management of civilian intra-articular gunshot wounds: treatment considerations and proposal of a classification system. Injury 29 [Suppl 1]:SA1–SA6

40. Gautier E, Stutz P (1994) Combination of the small external fixator and standard tubular system. Injury 25 [Suppl 4]:35–38

41. Graham TJ, Fitzgerald MS (2000) The destroyed elbow. Am J Orthop 29:9–15

42. Gugala Z, Lindsey RW (2003) Classification on gunshot injuries in civilians. Clin Orthop 408:65–81

43. Gur E, Atesalp S, Basbozkurt M et al (1999) Treatment of complex calcaneal fractures with bone defects from land mine blast injuries with a circular external fixator. Foot Ankle Int 20:37–41

44. Gustilo RB (1990) Current concepts review: the management of open fractures. J Bone Joint Surg 72A:299–304

45. Gustilo RB, Mendoza RM, Williams DN (1984) Problems in the management of type III (severe) open fractures: a new classification of type III open fractures. J Trauma 24:742–746

46. Hadziahmetovic Z, Gavrankapetanovc F, Masic I (1999) Dilemmas in the classification of foot injuries caused by land mines. Med Arch 53:65–66

47. Haidukewych GJ (2002) Temporary external fixation for the management of complex intra- and periarticular fractures of the lower extremity. J Orthop Trauma 16:678–685

48. Hammer RR, Rooser B, Lidman D et al (1996) Simplified external fixation for primary management of severe musculoskeletal injuries under war and peace time condition. J Orthop Trauma 10:545–554

49. Hammert WC, Minarchek J, Trzeciak MA (2000) Free-flap reconstruction of traumatic lower extremity wounds. Am J Orthop 29:22–26

50. Hansen S (1989) Overview of the severely traumatized lower limb. Reconstruction versus amputation. Clin Orthop 243:17–19

51. Harwood PJ, Giannoudis PV, Probst C et al (2006) The risk of local infective complications after damage control procedures for femoral shaft fracture. J Orthop Trauma 20:181–189

52. Hawkins BJ, Langerman RJ, Anger DM et al (1994) The Ilizarov technique in ankle fusion. Clin Orthop 303:217–225

53. Henley MB, Chapman JR, Agel J et al (1998) Treatment of type II, IIIA, and IIIB open fractures of the tibial shaft: A prospective comparison of unreamed interlocking intramedullary nails and half-pin external fixators. J Orthop Trauma 12:1–7

54. Herscovici D, Sanders RW, Scaduto J et al (2003) Vacuum assisted wound closure (VAC therapy) for the management of patients with high-energy soft tissue injuries. J Orthop Trauma 17:683–688

55. Holmes G (2003) Gunshot wounds of the foot. Clin Orthop 408:86–91

56. Hopkinson DAW, Marshall TK (1967) Fire-arm injuries. Br J Surg 54:344–353

57. Ilizarov GA (1992) Pseudoarthrosis and defect of long tubular bones. In: Transosseous osteosynthesis. Springer, Berlin Heidelberg New York

58. Johnson E, Strauss E (2003) Recent advantages in the treatment of gunshot fractures of the humeral shaft. Clin Orthop 408:126–132

59. Johnson EE, Weltmer J, George JL et al (1992) Ilizarov ankle arthrodesis. Clin Orthop 280:160–169

60. Karas EH, Strauss E, Sohail S (1995) Surgical stabilization of humeral shaft fractures due to gunshot wounds. Orthop Clin North Am 26:65–73

61. Keating J, Simpson A, Robinson C (2005) The management of fractures with bone loss. J Bone Joint Surg 87B:142–150

62. Kenwright J, Richardson JB, Goodship AE et al (1986) Effect of controlled axial micromovement on healing of tibial fractures. Lancet 2:1185–1187

63. Kenwright J, Richardson JB, Cunningham JL et al (1991) Axial movement and tibial fractures: a controlled randomized trial of treatment. J Bone Joint Surg 73B:654–659

64. Khalily C, Voor MJ, Seligson D (1998) Fracture site motion with Ilizarov and hybrid external fixation. J Orthop Trauma 12:21–26

65. Khouri RK (1992) Avoiding free flap failure. Clin Plast Surg 19:773–781

66. Kline DG, Hackett ER, Happel LH (1986) Surgery for lesions of the brachial plexus. Arch Neurol 43:170–181

67. Knight SL (1999) Open tibial fractures: principles of soft tissue cover. Curr Orthop 13:92–98

68. Labeeu F, Pasuch M, Toussaint P et al (1996) External fixation in war traumatology: report from the Rwandese war (October 1, 1990 to August 1, 1993). J Trauma 40: S223–S227

69. Lerner A, Solomenko A (1990) The alloplasty of a subtotal defect of the first metacarpal bone during the primary surgical treatment of a wound. Zdravoochranenie Belorussii 9:48

70. Lerner A, Soudry M (2003) Treatment of severe complicated bilateral lower extremity fractures according to Ilizarov method. Traumatol Orthopaedy Russia 1:5–8

71. Lerner A, Stein H (2004) Hybrid thin wire external fixation: an effective, minimal invasive, modular surgical tool for the stabilization of periarticular fractures. Orthopaedics 27:59–62

72. Lerner A, Freiman S, Nierenberg G et al (1998) External fixation frame extension for pressure sore prevention. Injury 29:730–731

73. Lerner A, Nierenberg G, Stein H (1998) Ilizarov external fixation in the management of bilateral, highly complex blast injuries of lower extremities: a report of two cases. J Orthop Trauma 12:442–445

74. Lerner A, Stahl S, Stein H (2000) Hybrid external fixation in high energy elbow fractures. A modular system with a promising future. J Trauma 49:1017–1022

75. Lerner A, Ullmann Y, Stein H et al (2000) Using the Ilizarov external fixation device for skin expansion. Ann Plast Surg 45:535–537

76. Lerner A, Weisz I, Nierenberg G et al (2000) Management of compound high energy injuries of the limbs. Harefuah 138:283–286

77. Lerner A, Hörer D, Merom L et al (2003) Modular use of external fixation configurations for treatment of complex and severely injured limbs. Eur J Trauma 29:108–111

78. Lerner A, Rosen N, Stahl S et al (2003) Treatment of severe gunshot fractures of the elbow region using the Ilizarov technique. Genij Ortopedii 2:41–45

79. Lerner A, Fodor L, Soudry M et al (2004) Acute shortening – modular treatment modality for severe combined bone and soft tissue loss of the extremities. J Trauma 57:603–608

80. Lerner A, Stein H, Soudry M (2004) Compound high-energy limb fractures with delayed union: our experience with adjuvant ultrasound stimulation (exogen). Ultrasonics 42:915–917

81. Lerner A, Chezar A, Haddad M et al (2005) Complications encountered while using thin-wire-hybrid-external fixation modular frames for fracture fixation. A retrospective clinical analysis and possible support for Damage Control Orthopaedic Surgery. Injury 36:590–598

82. Lerner A, Fodor L, Stein H et al (2005) Extreme bone lengthening using distraction osteogenesis after trauma. J Orthop Trauma 19:420–424

83. Lerner A, Stein H, Calif E (2005) Unilateral, hinged external fixation frame for elbow compression arthrodesis: the stepwise attainment of a stable 90-degree flexion position. A case report. J Orthop Trauma 19:52–55

84. Lerner A, Fodor L, Soudry M (2006) Is staged external fixation a valuable strategy for war injuries to the limbs? Clin Orthop Relat Res 448:217–224

85. Levin LS, Goldner RD, Urbaniak JR et al (1990) Management of severe musculoskeletal injuries of the upper extremity. J Orthop Trauma 4:432–440

86. Liebergall M, Segal D, Peyser A et al (1999) Combined injuries to the lower limbs. Injury 30:29–33

87. Liu Y, Chen X, Chen SLX et al (1988) Wounding effects of small fragments of different shapes at different velocities on soft tissues of dogs. J Trauma 28:S95–S98

88. Long W, Chang W, Brien E (2003) Grading system for gunshot injuries to the femoral diaphysis in civilians. Clin Orthop 408:92–100

89. Lowenberg DW, Feibel RJ, Louie KW et al (1996) Combined muscle flap and Ilizarov reconstruction for bone and soft tissue defects. Clin Orthop 332:37–51

90. MacKenzie EJ, Bosse MJ, Kellam JF et al (2002) Factors influencing the decision to amputate or reconstruct after high-energy lower extremity trauma. J Trauma 52:641–649

91. Martin RR, Byrne M (1977) Postoperative care and complications of damage control surgery. Surg Clin North Am 77:929–942

92. McAndrew MP, Lantz BA (1989) Initial care of massively traumatized lower extremities. Clin Orthop Relat Res 243:20–29

93. McHale KA, Gajewski DA (2002) The floating ankle: a pattern of violent injury. Treatment with thin-pin external fixation. Mil Med 167:454–458

94. Melcher GA, Hauke C, Metzdorf A et al (1996) Infection after intramedullary nailing: an experimental investigation on rabbits. Injury 27:SC23–SC26

95. Meyer JP, Lim LT, Schuler JJ et al (1985) Peripheral vascular trauma from close-range shotgun injuries. Arch Surg 120:1126–1131

96. Moed BR, Fakhouri AJ (1991) Compartment syndrome after low-velocity gunshot wounds to the forearm. J Orthop Trauma 5:134–137

97. Morykwas MJ, Argenta LC, Shelton-Brown EI et al (1997) Vacuum assisted closure: a new method for wound control and treatment. Animal studies and basic foundation. Ann Plast Surg 38:553–561

98. Nanobashvili J, Kopadze T, Tvaladze M et al (2003) War injuries of major extremity arteries. World J Surg 27:134–139

99. Nechaev EA, Grizanov AI, Fomin NF et al (1994) Mine-blast injuries [in Russian]. Ald, St. Petersburg, p 488

100. Nicolic D, Jovanovic Z, Popovic Z et al (1999) Primary surgical treatment of war injuries of major joints of limbs. Injury 30:129–134

101. Nork SE (2005) Initial fracture management and results. J Orthop Trauma 19:S7–S10

102. Norris BI, Kellam JF (1997) Soft-tissue injuries associated with high-energy extremity trauma: principles of management. J Am Acad Orthop Surg 5:37–46

103. Omer GE (1974) Injuries to nerves of the upper extremity. J Bone Joint Surg 56A:1615–1624

104. Paley D (2002) Principles of deformity correction. Springer, Berlin Heidelberg New York

105. Pape HC, Grimme K, Van Griensven M et al (2003) EFFORT Study Group. Impact of intramedullary instrumentation versus damage control for femoral fractures on immunoinflammatory parameters: prospective randomized analysis by the EFFORT Study Group. J Trauma 55:7–13

106. Parisien JS, Esformes I (1984) The role of arthroscopy in the management of low-velocity gunshot wounds of the knee joint. Clin Orthop 185:207–213

107. Reis ND, Dolev E (1989) Manual of disaster medicine. Springer, Berlin Heidelberg New York, p 475

108. Reis ND, Zinman C, Besser MIB et al (1991) A philosophy of limb salvage in war. Use of the fixateur externe. Mil Med 156:505–520

109. Ricci WM (2005) Comments on Egol KA et al., Staged management of high-energy proximal tibia fractures (OTA types 41). The results of the prospective standardized protocol. J Orthop Trauma 19:456

110. Ring D, Jupiter JB (1999) Mangling upper limb injuries in industry. Injury 30:B5–B13

111. Rozbruch SR, Wetzman AM, Watson JT et al (2006) Simultaneous treatment of tibial bone and soft tissue defects with the Ilizarov method. J Orthop Trauma 20:197–205

112. Salam AA, Eyres KS, Cleary J et al (1991) The use of a tourniquet when plating tibial fractures. J Bone Joint Surg Br 73:86–87

113. Sarmiento A, Zagorski JB, Zych GA et al (2000) Functional bracing for the treatment of fractures of the humeral diaphysis. J Bone Joint Surg 82A:478–486

114. Shepherd L, Zalavras C, Jaki K et al (2003) Gunshot femoral shaft fractures: is the current classification system reliable? Clin Orthop 408:101–109

115. Simpson B, Wilson R, Grant R (2003) Antibiotic therapy in gunshot injuries. Clin Orthop 408:82–85

116. Sinclair JS, McNally MA, Small JO et al (1997) Primary free-flap cover of open tibial fractures. Injury 28:581–586

117. Smith DK, Cooney WP (1990) External fixation of high-energy upper extremity injuries. J Orthop Trauma 4:7–18

118. Solomenko A, Lerner A, Truchan A (1981) The experience of using skin autoplasty after Krasovitov. Vestnik Chirurgii 9:90–91

119. Solomin LN (2005) General aspects of transosseous osteosynthesis by Ilizarov apparatus [in Russian]. Morsar, St. Petersburg, p 544

120. Stahl S, Lerner A, Kaufman T (1999) Immediate autografting of bone in open fractures with bone loss of the hand: a preliminary report. Scand J Plast Reconstr Surg Hand Surg 33:117–122

121. Starker H, Volpin G, Lerner A et al (1999) Ilizarov reconstructive surgery in complex problems of the musculoskeletal system. Harefuah 136:182–190

122. Stein H, Horesh Z, Lerner A (2006) Current trends for the biological treatment of segmental bone loss in high-energy long bone fractures. Orthopedics 29:773–777

123. Stein H, Lerner A (2001) Advances in the treatment of chronic osteomyelitis. Current Orthopaedics 15:451–456

124. Stein H, Lerner A (2005) Is rigid fixation of the fibula indicated in tibial plafond fractures? Orthopedics 28:438

125. Stein H, Weize I, Hoerer D et al (1999) Musculoskeletal trauma: high- and low-energy injuries. Orthopedics 22:965–967

126. Stein H, Rozen N, Lerner A et al (2003) Minimally invasive surgical techniques for the reconstruction of calcaneal fractures. Orthopedics 26:1053–1056

127. Stewart MP, Kinninmonth A (1993) Shotgun wounds of the limbs. Injury 24:667–670

128. Stock W, Hierner R (1994) Treatment of the soft tissues in combined injuries to the bone and soft tissue. Injury 25:SA46–SA58

129. Swan KG, Swan RC (1989) Gunshot wounds: pathophysiology and management. Year Book Medical, Chicago

130. Swiontkowsky M (1989) Criteria for bone debridement in massive lower limb trauma. Clin Orthop 243:41–47

131. Switz D, Elmorshidy M, Deyerle W (1976) Bullets, joints and lead intoxication. A remarkable and instructive case. Arch Intern Med 136:939–941

132. Tan V, Daluiski A, Capo J et al (2005) Hinged elbow external fixators: indications and uses. J Am Acad Orthop Surg 13:503–514

133. Tejan J, Lindsey R (1998) Management of civilian gunshot injuries of the femur. A review of the literature. Injury 29:18–22

134. Tejwani NC, Achan P (2004) Staged management of high-energy proximal tibial fractures. Bull Hos Jt Dis 62:62–66

135. Tscherne H, Regel G (1996) Care of the polytraumatised patient. J Bone Joint Surg Br 78(5):840–852

136. Tull F, Borrelli J (2003) Soft-tissue injury associated with closed fractures: evaluation and management. J Am Acad Orthop Surg 11:431–438

137. Ullmann Y, Lerner A, Ramon Y et al (2000) Interdigital bridging for treatment of the burned hand. Ann Burns Fire Disasters 13:92–93

138. Ullmann Y, Fodor L, Ramon Y et al (2006) The revised reconstructive ladder and its applications for high-energy injuries to the extremities. Ann Plast Surg Apr 56:401–405

139. Van-Raay JJ, Raaymakers EL, Dupree HW (1991) Knee ligament injuries combined with ipsilateral femoral and tibial fractures: the floating knee. Arch Orthop Trauma Surg 110:75–77

140. Watson JT, Moed BR, Karges DE et al (2000) Pilon fractures. Treatment protocol based on severity of soft tissue injury. Clin Orthop 375:78–90

141. Weitz-Marshall A, Bosse M (2002) Timing of closure of open fractures. J Am Acad Orthop Surg 10:379–384

142. Wightman JM, Gladish SL (2001) Explosions and blast injuries. Ann Emerg Med 37:664–678

143. Williams TM, Marsh JL, Nepola JV et al (1998) External fixation of tibial plafond fractures: is routine plating of the fibula necessary? J Orthop Trauma 12:16–20

144. Wilson R (2003) Gunshots to the hand and upper extremity. Clin Orthop 408:133–144

145. Wisniewski TF, Radziejowski MJ (1996) Gunshot fractures of the humeral shaft treated with external fixation. J Orthop Trauma 10:273–278

146. Zalavras C, Patzakis M (2003) Open fractures: evaluation and management. J Am Acad Orthop Surg 11:212–219

147. Zinman C, Norman D, Hamoud K, Reis ND (1997) External fixation for severe open fractures of the humerus caused by missiles. J Orthop Trauma 11(7):536–539

148. Ziperman HH (1961) The management of soft tissue missile wounds in war and peace. J Trauma 1:361–367

149. Zura R, Bosse M (2003) Current treatment of gunshot wounds to the hip and pelvis. Clin Orthop 408:110–114

Subject Index